Heartburn Cured

The Low Carb Miracle

Norm Robillard, Ph.D.

The information presented in this book is not intended as medical advice or as a substitute for consultations with your primary care physician. This information should be used in conjunction with the advice of your own doctor. Consult your doctor before initiating any diet. Your doctor is in a position to know about any medical conditions that you may have as well as any medication or supplements you may be taking. This diet plan should not be used by patients on dialysis.

Heartburn Cured: The Low Carb Miracle. Copyright © 2005 by Norm Robillard, Ph.D. All rights reserved. Printed in the United States of America. No part of this book may be used or reproduced in any manner what-so-ever without written permission, except in the case of brief quotations embodied in critical articles or reviews. For information, write to Heartburn Cured at P.O. Box 1685 Thousand Oaks CA 91360-4343. To purchase additional copies of this book, visit the web site Heartburncured.com.

Cover photo; Norm Robillard
Cover design; Peter Radford

ISBN 0-9766425-0-6

This book is dedicated to my son and daughter in law, John and Shannon Robillard for convincing me to experiment with reduced carbohydrate dieting.

Contents

ACKNOWLEDGMENTS V

Introduction 1

Chapter 2 Heartburn and GERD 13

Chapter 3 Current Treatments 23

Chapter 4 Human Digestion 35

Chapter 5 A New Theory 55

Chapter 6 My GERD Friendly Diet 88

Index 125

Acknowledgments

I want to thank my younger son Joseph Robillard for contributing to the research in this book. I am grateful to my parents, Norm and Martha Robillard for their support and encouragement.

The editorial feedback provided by Janet Garufis, John Patti and Kathy McCartney is greatly appreciated. Kathy McCartney also drew figure 1.

I want to acknowledge my grandson Tyler for reminding me daily of the power of curiosity.

Introduction

Things sweet to taste prove in digestion sour.
William Shakespeare

Heartburn is the most common symptom of gastroesophageal reflux disease (GERD), a condition that affects more than 60 million Americans and countless more across the globe. According to the Food and Drug Administration (FDA), more than one third of those afflicted with GERD suffer from daily symptoms. GERD seriously impacts both the health and quality of life of those who suffer from it. This book proposes a dramatic new approach for controlling GERD developed by a microbiologist (me) who suffered extensively with GERD and can speak first hand of the symptoms as well as a dramatic new and effective approach that turns conventional wisdom and medical doctrine on its head. In writing this book I have two goals: 1. Describe my theory that the consumption of excess dietary carbohydrates is the root cause of GERD in susceptible individuals. 2. Put my theory into action tailoring low carbohydrate dieting to individuals with chronic heartburn. This book will help people with GERD maintain a normal healthy diet while reducing carbohydrate consumption enough to alleviate the symptoms of acid reflux.

I am not surprised that the true cause of GERD has remained a mystery for so long. The significant amount of misinformation on this subject is mind-boggling. Those seeking relief from heartburn are advised to stop smoking, refrain from consuming alcohol, avoid coffee, reduce fatty foods, avoid lying down, eat less, avoid "trigger foods" and loosen clothing. If that does not work, there are over-the-counter and prescription medicines that block the production of stomach acid that is needed to digest food. If you still have symptoms, you can even undergo a variety of radical surgeries.

The problem with current heartburn advice is that it is often wrong or misleading and simply does not work. Acid reducing medicines, at best, offer partial and temporary relief, are not intended for chronic use and are associated with side effects and health risks. According to a report in the Journal of the American Medical Association (1), "Current use of gastric acid-suppressive therapy was associated with an increased risk of community-acquired pneumonia." One heartburn medicine was withdrawn from the market because of reported deaths.

This book introduces my groundbreaking theory about the root cause of GERD and a dramatically different approach to control this disease by attacking the underlying cause of acid reflux. This approach has already cured many GERD sufferers including me. The simple truth is that the consumption of excess carbohydrates is the main cause of GERD and the cure is a reduced carbohydrate, high protein, high fat (that's right, high fat) diet. Low carbohydrate dieting has already been credited with preventing and even reversing type II diabetes, coronary heart disease, high blood pressure, and obesity. So get ready to throw away your antacids and acid reducers and say goodbye once and for all to heartburn. My low carb approach is the most effective treatment for heartburn available, will improve your overall health, and allow you to control your weight as well. This diet is more flexible than the other low carb diets and allows for cheating. It's not really cheating, but rather adjusting your carbohydrate levels in response to your symptoms.

My Own Heartburn Journey

As an adult, during my 20 years of research and drug development in the pharmaceutical industry, I have been plagued, like so many people, with chronic heartburn caused by GERD. Even though I was taking acid reducers and antacids, my condition continued to get worse. On a business trip to Seattle in the fall of 2003, after arriving at my hotel, I ate dinner and retired to my room. I went to bed at about 11:00 PM, as I was to attend an all day meeting the next day before flying home. I awoke in the middle of the night and leapt out of bed, still half dreaming, and thinking, "Oh my god, this is what it feels like to die." I couldn't breathe; I was choking for air and my lungs felt like they were filled with burning liquid. I ran to the bathroom coughing up something from my lungs that simply did not register. It felt like acid was in my lungs. I soon realized that I had suffered severe acid reflux; stomach acid that traveled up my esophagus until I aspirated it into my lungs. I will never forget this moment. It defines the kind of fear and suffering that is possible with GERD.

A month or so after my trip to Seattle, having gained some weight, I decided to join my son, John, and daughter in-law,

Introduction

Shannon, in trying reduced carbohydrate dieting. I did not follow any specific low carb diet plan and continued to drink coffee and consume alcohol. Within one or two days after starting the diet, the chronic heartburn, I had suffered for more than 20 years, completely ceased. I was totally amazed and shocked. How could GERD, a chronic condition that had plagued me for so long, be cured so easily? I have not taken one single form of heartburn medication since.

I am happy to report that I no longer suffer at all with this ailment (except when I cheat, which I have done for fun and to test my theory). I never use heartburn medication of any kind because I don't need it. My symptoms are gone. How did this miraculous change take place? What caused the change? Had I eliminated some of the trigger foods mentioned in all the heartburn literature? I was still drinking coffee and drinking alcohol (wine and mixed drinks using diet cola only). It couldn't be the fats because fats make up the major energy source in low carb dieting and I was consuming significant amounts. Could it be that carbohydrates as an entire food group had been causing my heartburn all these years?

I Am Not Alone

While researching heartburn and low carbohydrate dieting, I realized that I was not alone. Many other people were claiming the same thing. That is, soon after reducing carbohydrates in their diet, numerous heartburn sufferers were reporting that their symptoms simply vanished. The Internet chat rooms and bulletin boards are filled with experiences of people reporting this amazing phenomenon. Do a simple search on GOOGLE to see for yourself. And it is not just ordinary people. Recently, physicians have now begun to realize the benefits of this approach for treating GERD patients and have alluded to this phenomenon in books such as "Protein Power." In this New York Times best selling book, Dr. Michael and Mary Dan Eades report on the alleviation of reflux as the "most predictable beneficial effects" of low carb dieting. The beneficial effect of controlling carbohydrates on GERD is also noted in the book "Akins for Life" by Dr. Robert Atkins.

A San Francisco, California based physician, Tom Cowan, wrote "I have used a low-carbohydrate approach for the treatment of GERD for many years and with many patients. I can report that it is one of the most effective interventions that I use. It is not unusual for people to report relief even within a few days." (2).

My research-based theory is also corroborated by a recent clinical study supporting the ability of low carb dieting to stop GERD (3). Five individuals are described in this case report. They all experienced a significant improvement in GERD symptoms after starting a low-carbohydrate diet. The results of this study suggest that carbohydrate restriction likely contributed to their symptom relief. This study was the first to suggest that certain foods such as coffee and fat may not matter when a low-carbohydrate diet is followed. You can bet that there will soon be additional studies with larger patient populations because the National Institute of Diabetes and Digestive and Kidney Diseases is making the funding available, stating: "The Committee is aware of new research which indicates a controlled carbohydrate diet may dramatically reduce the incidence of gastroesophageal reflux (heartburn)." But why wait? The low carb approach has so many other health benefits to offer as well as eliminating heartburn.

Of Men (And Women) and Microbes

Feeling encouraged by my preliminary reading, I began researching in earnest how a reduced carbohydrate diet could stop chronic acid reflux. I wanted to understand what the carbohydrates could be doing or what properties they possessed that seemed to contribute to heartburn. As I began to study human digestion of carbohydrates, proteins and fats, I immediately realized that my effort would need to explore not only the human digestive process, but also the role of microorganisms in digestion. Microbes are normally present in our intestinal tract and play a significant role in digestion. Microbial populations in our intestines are mostly bacteria and are considered friendly inhabitants providing vitamins and other essential nutrients our bodies need yet cannot make.

A few important facts from my early education in medical microbiology immediately came to mind. The intestines are anaerobic, for the most part, meaning that there is very little oxygen present. Intestinal microorganisms need to process nutrients and gain energy by a process called fermentation (food breakdown in the absence of oxygen); where as the cells in our body typically use aerobic respiration and can metabolize nutrients with the help of oxygen. These two metabolic pathways (fermentation and respiration) are very different yet both play a significant role in how food is broken down and utilized. And anyone who has made beer or wine knows fermentation means lots and lots of gas. It was not too long before I had a clear working theory.

> Excess dietary carbohydrates escape absorption by our intestines. Microbes breakdown these carbohydrates quickly producing gas and acid as end products. The resulting gas creates intestinal pressure, which is the driving force for acid reflux. Less gas is produced by the microbial breakdown of fats and proteins and therefore consumption of excess carbohydrates, but not proteins and fats, will result in heartburn in susceptible individuals.

To offer a better understanding of my theory I need to set the stage. This book reviews and explains heartburn and other symptoms and conditions caused by GERD, the diagnosis of GERD and drugs, and other remedies, including surgery, aimed at treating this condition. I challenge the current theory that "spontaneous relaxations" of the lower esophageal sphincter are responsible for this condition. I explain the human digestive process and describe the basic structure and properties carbohydrates, proteins and fats, the three main food groups comprising our diet. I also explain how these three food groups are processed not only by our own digestive system, but how our friendly gut inhabitants, the microbes, depend on these very same foods. As these discussions come together, you will see how consuming carbohydrates is a lot like burning gas in a diesel engine. Carbs burn fast (the microbes metabolize them quickly releasing gas), while fats and proteins burn slow (the microbes metabolize them more slowly producing less gas). For susceptible individuals like me and 60 million other men, women and children in the USA alone, the result is heartburn. A second key part of this book puts this information into action. I provide important dietary information that tailors low carb dieting to individuals with heartburn. I provide a clear strategy for meal planning to help you cure your heartburn once and for all.

My unique experience with GERD, my passion for a cure, and my professional background position me well to write this book. I have studied and published my research on

Introduction

human gut microorganisms as a postdoctoral fellow at Tufts University in Boston. Over the last twenty-five years I have conducted research on numerous microorganisms including the prevalent gut microorganism *Bacteroides fragilis,* methacillin-resistant *Staphylococcus aureus, Bacillus anthracis, Pseudomonas aeruginosa, Escherchia coli* and several viruses. I have worked for both pharmaceutical and biotechnology companies developing medicines to improve human health. My work has been published in peer review journals, national meeting abstracts and books. My honest and factual evaluation of a low carb approach to treating this disease is supported with numerous journal references, my own experiences, and experiences of well-known physicians and the success stories of other people. I believe this book will benefit patients, doctors and nurses as well as private and public researchers in the field of gastrointestinal research.

People want answers and solutions that do not involve expensive and risky drugs, invasive procedures and confusing and misleading advice. The message I deliver is simple. Reduce your intake of carbohydrates. If you are like most heartburn sufferers, you will experience a rapid elimination of your symptoms.

References

1. Laheij RJ, Sturkenboom MC, Hassing RJ, Dieleman J, Stricker BH, Jansen JB. Risk of community-acquired pneumonia and use of gastric acid-suppressive drugs. JAMA. 2004 Oct 27; 292 (16):1955-60.

2. Cowan T, Wise Traditions in Food, Farming and the Healing Arts, the quarterly magazine of the Weston A. Price Foundation, Winter 2002.

3. Yancy, WS Jr, Provenzale D, Westman EC, Improvement of gastroesophageal reflux disease after initiation of a low-carbohydrate diet: five brief case reports, Altern Ther Health Med, 2001, Nov-Dec; 7 (6): 120, 116-9

Chapter 2

Heartburn and GERD – What is it?

"Indigestion is the failure to adjust a square meal to a round stomach."

Unknown

This chapter focuses on describing Gastroesophageal Reflux Disease (GERD), the symptoms and complications of the disease, and current theory on the cause of GERD.

Heartburn

If you are reading this book, heartburn symptoms are likely well known to you, or someone you care about. Symptoms can include intense burning in the chest behind the breastbone, small regurgitations and extreme discomfort. Heartburn is thought to be caused by stomach acid backing up into the esophagus. Actually, heartburn can be caused not only by the reflux of stomach contents (acid) into the esophagus, but reflux of intestinal contents including bile from the duodenum (the upper part of your small intestine that connects to the stomach).

As shown in Figure 1, the esophagus is a tube that connects your mouth to your stomach. The tube is surrounded by muscles that contract in concert to keep food moving towards the stomach once swallowed. This swallowing process is called peristalsis. What normally keeps food in the stomach once it arrives is the lower esophageal sphincter (LES). The LES consists of several muscles that encircle the esophagus above the stomach that open, or relax, as food

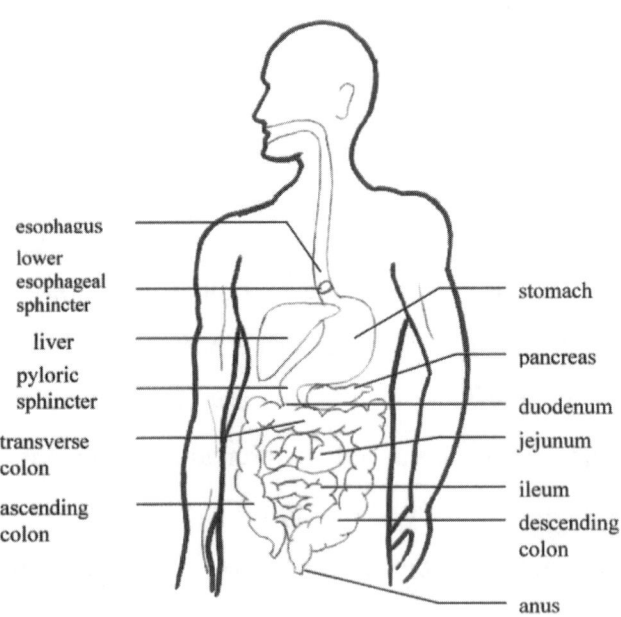

Figure1. Human digestive system

approaches and then reseal. Heartburn results when the LES does not stay closed allowing the contents of the stomach including hydrochloric acid (HCL) and duodenal contents, back into the esophagus. The pain from heartburn is caused because the esophagus does not have the same protective mucous that the stomach has and the acid and duodenal contents like bile "burn" the unprotected tissue.

GERD

Mild and occasional heartburn is fairly common, but more frequent heartburn or more severe symptoms generally result in a diagnosis of GERD or Gastroesophageal Reflux Disease. While many more definitive tests[1] can confirm the diagnosis and assess damage to the esophagus, the initial diagnosis is usually based on the patient's history including the frequency and severity of heartburn and other related symptoms. GERD is as common in women as in men (1). There are several definitions of GERD but the most common one is "Symptoms and or tissue injury resulting from the reflux of gastric (stomach) contents into the esophagus" (American Society of Gastrointestinal Endoscopy).

The leading theory on the cause of GERD is that lower esophageal sphincter muscles (that normally provide a barrier between your stomach and esophagus) are weaker in GERD patients and that these muscles relax spontaneously in GERD patients allowing stomach contents to escape into the esophagus. The phenomenon has been termed "transient relaxation of the lower esophageal sphincter" or TRLES. This theory is widely accepted as the underlying cause of GERD. Later on in this book, I will contrast current theory with my own theory that gas produced by microorganisms in our intestinal tract is the true cause of GERD and by limiting carbohydrates in our diets we can prevent the microbes from producing as much gas.

1. Tests used to assess esophageal damage and confirm diagnosis of GERD. 1. pH studies the acidity of the lower esophagus is measured continually. 2. Esophagoscopy procedures involve visually examining the inside of the esophagus. 3. Manometry measures the pressure of the lower esophageal sphincter muscle. 4. X-rays of swallowed barium can monitor food flow between the esophagus and stomach.

Other Symptoms

Heartburn is the most common complaint associated with GERD but there are other symptoms associated with reflux that include a sour taste, belching, regurgitation, sore throat, hoarseness, laryngitis (remember the Ashley Simpson Saturday Night Live lip syncing story) painful swallowing, persistent cough, asthma, gingivitis, dental erosion, bad breath, and earaches. I personally have experienced chronic coughing associated with GERD. I was prescribed prescription strength acid reducing medicine because the over the counter medication I was taking was not strong enough. Prior to writing this book, I had no idea how common this symptom is and given the pulmonary complications that can arise (see Complications of GERD) this symptom deserves special mention.

As I researched more about GERD, I found some interesting statistics on chronic cough. In a recent study of seventy-eight patients who complained of cough 41% were found to have GERD as a contributing cause. Only asthma (59 %) and postnasal drip syndrome (58 %) were more frequent contributing causes (2). I find these results amazing and wonder if GERD is being under diagnosed due to the variety symptoms, some of which are not recognized or reported, that relate to underlying GERD.

Complications of GERD

In addition to the primary symptoms of GERD, there are many secondary complications associated with GERD, some of which are extreme and even life threatening. Repeated GER episodes can result in permanent injury to the esophagus. This scarring can lead to a narrowing of the esophagus referred to as a stricture. This narrowing results in a condition called dysphagia, where swallowing is affected. Dysphagia can be described as the sensation of food getting stuck in the esophagus after swallowing and often indicates an advanced stage of esophageal damage. What we are talking about here is difficulty or even the inability to swallow. I cannot imagine what that must feel like.

Barrett's syndrome

Over time, untreated gastroesophageal reflux may lead to the development of Barrett's esophagus. Barrett's esophagus is a pre-cancerous condition that begins in the lower esophagus where once normal cells lining the esophagus change into a cell type that resembles cells of the stomach. This occurs as a result of esophageal damage from continued acid reflux. Barrett's esophagus may be suspected by endoscopic evaluation of the esophagus, but the diagnosis is confirmed by endoscopically biopsied tissue (3). Barrett's esophagus can, in rare cases, progress to adenocarcinoma (cancer that develops in the esophagus).

Lung Injury Caused by GERD

Gastroesophageal reflux can lead to chronic, severe lung damage and recurrent infections. Lung injury is caused by the reflux of stomach acid and other intestinal juices into the lungs. Aspiration of gastric juice into the lungs can also lead to pulmonary fibrosis. Pulmonary fibrosis is a serious condition that can require lung transplantation.

Children and GERD

It may come as a surprise, that children (especially asthmatic children) are significantly impacted by this disease. GERD is a common cause of chronic cough in children. As many as 50% of children with chronic respiratory diseases have "silent" gastroesophageal reflux (GER) (4, 5). Left untreated, serious respiratory complications of GERD can include chronic bronchitis, exacerbation of asthma, and other lung diseases. Unfortunately, because GERD can be difficult to diagnose in the situation where the child does not exhibit the typical symptoms of GERD like heartburn, sour taste, or regurgitation, parents may be unaware of the danger of GERD. Many of these children once diagnosed, ultimately undergo surgery to address the condition (6).

If you have a child (older than a toddler) with severe GERD suffering from significant complications, check with your pediatrician about the advisability of lowering the carbohydrate levels in your child's diet. I do think lowering carb levels in your child's diet is worth looking into if your child is suffering from significant GERD related symptoms and is at risk for respiratory complications. I recently spoke with a friend who reported that his daughter, who suffered significantly with this disease from a very young age, had undergone surgery for her condition. To me, it seems reasonable to explore the potential benefits of a reduced carbohydrate diet in children suffering with GERD as an alternative to surgery (refer to surgery for GERD and related side effects in chapter 3). But, let me repeat myself here. Consult your pediatrician!

References
1. 1. Lin M, Gerson LB, Lascar R, Davila M, Triadafilopoulos G. Features of gastroesophageal reflux disease in women. Am J Gastroenterol. 2004. 99(8):1442-7.
2. A pathogenic triad in chronic cough - Asthma, postnasal drip syndrome, and gastroesophageal reflux disease (Palombini B.C.; Villanova C.A.C.; Araujo E.; Gastal O.L.; Alt D.C.; Stolz D.P.; Palombini C.O. Chest: 116. 79-84.
3. Shalauta, MD, Saad, R. American Family Physician. May 2004.
4. Juchet A, Bremont F, Dutau G, Olives JP. Chronic cough and gastroesophageal reflux in children Arch Pediatr. 2001 Aug; 8 Suppl 3:629-634.
5. Gorenstein A, Levine A, Boaz M, Mandelberg A, Serour F. Severity of acid gastroesophageal reflux assessed by pH metry: is it associated with

respiratory disease? Pediatr Pulmonol. 2003 Oct; 36(4): 330-4.

6. Mattioli G, Sacco O, Gentilino V, Martino F, Pini Prato A, Castagnetti M, Montobbio G, Jasonni V. Outcome of laparoscopic Nissen-Rossetti fundoplication in children with gastroesophageal reflux disease and supraesophageal symptoms. Surg Endosc. 2004 Mar; 18 (3): 463-5. Epub 2004 Feb 02.

Chapter 3

Treatments for GERD

"There are two kinds of light – the glow that illuminates and the glare that obscures."
James Thurber

In this chapter I review current treatment options for GERD sufferers as well as potential side effects and complications associated with each.

Diet

Several books and web-based guides have been published offering dietary approaches to control heartburn. As far as I am concerned, few, if any of them are worth the cover price. The book, "Tell Me What to Eat If I Have Acid Reflux," actually advises people with acid reflux to "Just say no to dieting" and instead recommends a wild array of high carbohydrate foods. Another book called "50 Ways to Relieve Heartburn" is informative in terms of the disease and diagnosis, but like virtually all the other heartburn books on the market, continues to push low fats / high carbs, the precise combination that results in GERD. A high fat diet does not cause GERD (1-3).

AstraZeneca, the pharmaceutical company that manufactures Nexium, an expensive prescription drug advertised for patients with chronic heartburn, promotes a meal plan "designed specifically to help you manage your GERD" that supplies over 275 grams of carbohydrates per day (you can find this meal plan on their Nexium website). For someone with GERD, that is a huge amount of carbohydrates to consume on a daily basis. Such a diet virtually ensures that heartburn sufferers will continue to consume more carbs than they can digest and absorb leaving plenty of leftovers for the microbes to produce gas from thus leading to more heartburn. This meal plan virtually assures that people susceptible to acid reflux will continue to require acid reducing drugs. I have come to understand that the only sound dietary advice for GERD is to reduce carbohydrate intake. If AstraZeneca was to offer my low carb diet plan on their web site I guarantee Nexium sales would drop dramatically.

Antacids

Antacids do exactly what their name implies; neutralize the acid in your stomach. Most people who have heartburn are very familiar with these over-the-counter products, such as Rolaids and Tums as well as simple bicarbonate. I have consumed my share. These over the counter medications reduce your stomach acid, but can have negative consequences long term. Because antacids cause the pH in the stomach to rise to a more neutral pH, the digestive enzyme pepsin that breaks down protein no longer functions. Above a pH of 4, pepsin activity ceases or is dramatically hindered. Because stomach acid forms a barrier between intestinal microbes and your stomach, esophagus and lungs, the reduction of stomach acidity, which results from taking antacids, makes you more susceptible to infections. So, even something as innocuous sounding as antacids, can potentially cause serious complications if used often or at high doses.

H2 Blockers

H2 blockers are one of the most commonly used medications for heartburn. Several H2 blockers are available over the counter (without a prescription). Tagamet (cimetidine), Pepcid (famotidine) and Zantac (ranitidine) were all used by me. These drugs block the normal production of hydrochloric acid by your stomach. The idea is to reduce the amount of acid in your stomach so even if you suffer reflux, there will be less acid to burn your esophagus.

Without going into too much detail, H2 blockers (also referred to as H2 receptor antagonists or HRAs) block your stomach's ability to produce acid. The "H" in H2 is for histamine. Histamine is the chemical messenger that tells your stomach to make acid when you smell food. HRAs block that message by binding to the same receptor that histamine does. The result is that parietal cells lining your stomach are not switched on and acid is not produced.

H2 blockers are generally taken once to twice per day but are not recommended for more than a couple of weeks without a visit to your doctor, a fact I learned while researching and writing this book. I literally lived on this medicine. I also learned that cimetidine has more drug interaction potential (so you need to be careful about taking other medications while on cimetidine) relative to the other drugs in this class.

The side effects for H2 blockers include constipation, diarrhea (interesting how the same drug can cause such opposite effects), headache, and in the case of cimetidine, breast enlargement, fatigue and impotence. Confusion and dizziness are side effects of the H2 blockers particularly in the elderly. The key message is that H2-blocker drugs, though widely promoted, are not indicated for long term use, have side effects and inhibit stomach acid that is essential for normal digestion.

Proton Pump Inhibitors

Proton Pump Inhibitors (PPIs), like H2 blockers, block your stomach's ability to produce acid. Drugs in this class include Prilosec (omeprazole), Nexium (esomeprazole), Zoton (lansoprazole), Pariet (rabeprazole) and Protium (pantoprazole). Proton pump inhibitors are generally considered more potent than H2 blockers at reducing stomach acid. Instead of blocking histamine binding, PPIs inhibit the microscopic pumps (called proton pumps) that make the acid inside the parietal cells. These little proton pumps are known as gastric H+K+ATPases. In simple terms, these pumps make protons (H+) needed for stomach acid, also known as hydrochloric acid, or HCl. If you stop the action of these pumps, no more acid is produced.

The most common side effects of PPI drugs are headache, diarrhea, constipation, abdominal pain, nausea, and rash. Note that these drugs interact with other drugs, such as certain blood clotting, epilepsy and antifungal drugs and so can interfere with the action of those drugs. The long-term use of proton pump inhibitors can lead to stomach infections and pose an increased risk for pneumonia because they significantly reduce the production of stomach acid. Over prescribing PPIs is a particular problem in the elderly who are more susceptible to infection. According to The American Medical Directors Association, Caring for the Ages web-based publication; "proton pump inhibitors are often over prescribed in long-term care, disregarding published guidelines for their use".

Pneumonia Risk from PPIs and H2 Antagonist Drugs

One of the increased health risks associated with the PPI and H2 Antagonist drugs is due to the dramatic reduction in the production of stomach acid. People taking acid reducing drugs have an increased risk of pneumonia as documented in a recent journal article from the Oct. 27, 2004 issue of the Journal of the American Medical Association. This study of more than 364,000 people led by Robert J.F. Laheij at the University Medical Center St. Radboud in Nijmegen, Netherlands, found the risk of pneumonia was almost double for people taking proton-pump inhibitors for prolonged periods. The risk was almost two-thirds higher for those taking histamine antagonists, compared to people not taking such drugs. According to Laheij, one reason long-term use of both classes of drugs can increase the risk of infection is that acid kills bacteria in the stomach. Lowering stomach acid lets more bacteria survive in the stomach (and presumably reflux into the lungs). Bacteria are normal inhabitants of our intestines and are essential for our survival. While these bacteria are, for the most part considered "friendly", if they are allowed to move from the intestines into the stomach due to reducing stomach acidity, they are positioned to reflux into the esophagus and lungs where they can cause disease. That is what puts people on acid reducing medicines at risk for pneumonia.

Prokinetic Agents

Prokinetic or promotility agents like Metoclopramide and Cisapride work by increasing LES strength and encouraging emptying of food from the stomach. Current prokinetic agents are not a reasonable first or second choice treatment because they have shown limited efficacy, and their side-effect profile outweighs their benefits (4). Side effects include nausea, diarrhea and nervous system effects. In the case of Cisapride, it was withdrawn from the market because there were 341 reports of heart rhythm abnormalities and 80 deaths. This information is published on the FDA.gov web site.

Surgery

In cases where therapy with histamine-2 blockers or proton pump inhibitors (PPIs) doesn't succeed in controlling symptoms, surgery is a third option elected by a surprising number of people. This surgery is also common in children with GERD. Surgery for GERD, such as Nissen Fundoplication (the preferred surgical method), improves the barrier between the esophagus and stomach to prevent gastric and duodenal contents from entering the esophagus. In the Nissen Fundoplication procedure (named after Rudolf Nissen) the surgeon pulls the stomach up and around the esophagus and then secures it around the esophagus. Antireflux surgery evaluated for 355 patients showed that this type of surgery involves a risk of serious complications and even death (5). Antireflux surgery can be done via open surgery or laparoscopy (where several small incisions are made and ports for inserting surgical instruments and cameras are put in place. Laparoscopic fundoplication has been performed since 1991). Laparoscopy requires a significant level of skill because the procedure is technically challenging and there is a risk of serious complications (6).

A significant number of patients report new symptoms following fundoplication surgery. In one study 54 of 151 patients reported new symptoms following surgery. The symptoms included excessive gas, abdominal bloating, and dysphagia (difficulty swallowing). The quality of life was reported to be significantly lower in patients with these symptoms and as many as one third required continued medical therapy after the operation. (7). In another study of 109 patients that underwent laparoscopic antireflux surgery,

30 patients (36%) also reported post surgery symptoms that included bloating and diarrhea (8). In another study of 60 patients, 51 (93%) had recurrent gastrointestinal symptoms that included flatulence, early satiety (feeling full after eating), meteorism (stomach gas), inability to vomit, dysphagia, diarrhea, epigastric (upper stomach) pain and inability to belch (9).

Given what we know about surgical outcomes, I would absolutely advise surgery only as a last resort. Hopefully, after reading this book and implementing my low carb diet plan, the need for surgery will be eliminated.

References:

1. Penagini R, Mangano M, Bianchi PA. Effect of increasing the fat content but not the energy load of a meal on gasto-oesophageal reflux and lower oesophageal sphincter motor function. *Gut* 1998; 42:330–3.
2. Pehl C, Waizenhoefer A, Wendl B, et al. Effect of low and high fat meals on lower esophageal sphincter

motility and gastroesophageal reflux in healthy subjects. *Am J Gastroenterol* 1999; 94:1192–6.

3. Ruhl CE, Everhart JE. Overweight, but not high dietary fat intake, increases risk of gastroesophageal reflux disease hospitalization: the NHANES I Epidemiologic Followup Study. First National Health and Nutrition Examination Survey. *Ann Epidemiol* 1999; 9:424–35.

4. Tutuian R, Castell DO. Management of gastroesophageal reflux disease. Am J Med Sci. 2003 Nov; 326(5): 309-18.

5. Urschel JD. Complications of antireflux surgery. Am J Surg. 1993 Jul; 166(1):68-70.

6. Collet D, Cadiere GB. Conversions and complications of laparoscopic treatment of gastro-oesophageal reflux disease. Am J Surg 1995; 169: 622-626.

7. Vakil N, Shaw M, Kirby R.Clinical effectiveness of laparoscopic fundoplication in a U.S. community. Am J Med. 2003 Jan; 114(1):1-5.

8. Klaus A, Hinder RA, DeVault KR, Achem SR. Bowel dysfunction after laparoscopic antireflux surgery: incidence, severity, and clinical course. The

American Journal of Medicine, Volume 114, Issue 1, Pages 6 - 9.

9. Beldi G, Glattli A.Long-term gastrointestinal symptoms after laparoscopic Nissan fundoplication. Surg Laparosc Endosc Percutan Tech. 2002 Oct; 12(5): 316-9.

Chapter 4

Human Digestion

"A good reliable set of bowels is worth more to a man than any quantity of brains."
Henry Wheeler Shaw

In this chapter I will explain the structure, properties and importance of each of the three main food groups; carbohydrates, proteins and fats. I will also explain human digestion and how the digestive process functions in specific ways using unique enzymes, acid and bile to break down each of these three very different types of food.

Although I will be describing three food groups, carbohydrates, proteins and fats, only two of them, proteins and fats are essential in our diet. Carbohydrates are not required, in that glucose, the only carbohydrate that is required by our body, can be synthesized by the body without the necessity of including it in the diet. Keep this point in mind as we discuss the food groups and also as we move on to implement my dietary plan, which calls for reducing excess carbohydrates in your diet.

Humans are omnivorous, that is, we are able to eat a variety of food types such as vegetables, grains, meats and dairy products. To derive energy and building blocks (like fatty acids, amino acids and glucose) to maintain our bodies, food must be broken down into smaller pieces (usually single molecules) and absorbed by our body via the intestines. This process is referred to as digestion. Digestion of foods and the absorption of nutrients is key for maintaining good health. Our digestive system is incredibly efficient and has evolved several mechanisms to obtain the highest possible benefit from multiple food sources. The food groups we derive energy and building blocks from fall into three categories; proteins, fats and carbohydrates. The food and liquids we consume also contain other needed nutrients such as vitamins, minerals and water.

Carbohydrates (As a Group)

Foods such as fruits, vegetables, grains, pasta, flour, potatoes, pastries, candy, rice, sugar and breads are mostly carbohydrate. Carbohydrates (sugars, starches and fiber) contain carbon, hydrogen and oxygen. That's how they got their name. Glucose is the carbohydrate our cells prefer to use to derive energy. Most of the carbohydrates we consume are eventually broken down to glucose. Therefore, the primary role of carbohydrates in our diet is fuel. This is important, because the ability of carbohydrates serve as "quick" energy sources is precisely the reason that excess carbohydrates can result in heartburn. As you will see later, microorganisms also prefer carbohydrates as a rapid fuel source producing energy as well as gas.

Carbohydrate Structure

The basic carbohydrate unit is called a monosaccharide, the most common and important monosaccharide being glucose. Monosaccharides can link together forming disaccharides (two sugar units) or polysaccharides (multiple sugar units). Linkage of two glucose molecules forms the disaccharide maltose, the product of starch hydrolysis. Linkage of glucose and galactose forms lactose, the main sugar in milk. Yes, milk is loaded with carbohydrates; so don't pay attention to that old adage that milk will sooth your heartburn. The relief will only be temporary. Linkage of glucose and fructose forms sucrose, also known as table sugar. Basic sugar units can also link together to form more complex sugars called polysaccharides.

Carbohydrates (Starch)

The most common polysaccharides in the human diet are starches. Starches are prevalent in foods like flour, rice, potatoes, bread, pasta, and grains. Starch is the major form of stored carbohydrate in plants. Starches are typically composed of 1000 or more glucose units. Starch is a polysaccharide composed of a mixture of amylose, an essentially linear polysaccharide, and amylopectin, a highly branched polysaccharide. Natural starches contain some amylose, but mostly amylopectin. Both forms of starch are polymers of glucose meaning that starches are long chains of glucose. Starches containing amylopectin have more cross-linking between the glucose chains.

Carbohydrates (Fiber)

Fiber is also considered a carbohydrate. The fiber in our diet is mostly cellulose and is associated with plant stems like celery but is also prevalent in oats, wheat and bran. Like amylose, fiber is an unbranched polysaccharide of glucose.

In this case, the long chains of glucose are not digestible by humans because we lack the enzymes necessary to break the bonds between the glucose units in fiber. Fiber forms the roughage in our diet and is considered "colon healthy".

The message is that carbohydrates (other than fiber) serve as fuel sources that can be broken down quickly and used for energy. This is the same property that leads to heartburn in susceptible individuals when carbohydrates are consumed in excess. As you will see in chapter 6, when implementing my no heartburn diet, the starchy carbohydrates derived from grains and the products made from them need to be limited. Also on the limited list, are sugars, the one and two unit carbohydrates like sucrose, fructose, maltose and lactose.

Proteins

Foods like meats, poultry, fish, eggs, whey and cheese are mostly protein but also contain fats. Protein can also be found in foods like nuts, soybeans and seeds. Proteins contain carbon, hydrogen, sulfur, oxygen and nitrogen. Proteins are generally large macromolecules that are composed of individual building blocks called amino acids. Amino acids have a different structure than the sugar units that make up carbohydrates. One important difference is that amino acids contain nitrogen and sulfur. This is one reason we cannot survive without protein. We need the nitrogen and sulfur to make our own proteins. Carbohydrates and fats do not contain nitrogen and sulfur.

The amino acids in proteins are used to make new proteins in our body including muscle cells (both heart and skeletal muscle), repair damaged cells and make enzymes and hormones. Many people do not realize that some of the amino acids in proteins can be used to synthesize glucose and this process occurs regularly in our body. So, as I mentioned earlier, our bodies do not actually require carbohydrates, since the basic unit of usable carbohydrate, glucose, can be made directly from proteins and used for energy.

Some amino acids can be made by our body (non essential amino acids) while others cannot (essential amino acids) and must either be provided in our diet or be supplied by friendly microorganisms living in our intestinal tract. Table 1 lists essential vs. non-essential amino acids. This information is generally not critical because most people consume a variety of proteins that would normally supply all of the essential amino acids. A problem could only arise on a protein restricted diet or general starvation.

Table 1. Essential vs. Non Essential Amino Acids

Essential Amino Acids	**Non Essential Amino Acids**
Arginine	Alanine
Histidine	Asparagine
Isoleucine	Aspartate
Leucine	Cysteine
Lysine	Glutamate
Methionine	Glutamine
Phenylalanine	Glycine
Threonine	Proline
Tryptophan	Serine
Valine	Tyrosine

Protein Structure

To form proteins, amino acids are linked together via peptide bonds. The peptide bonds form the backbone of the protein, which can be thought of as a long chain. There are 20 different amino acids that compose proteins. Proteins range in size from about 40 amino acids (smaller proteins are referred to as peptides) to hundreds of amino acids. The sequence of the amino acids in the protein chain determine its primary structure but the proteins fold back onto themselves in such a way as to have secondary and tertiary structure. The "refolded" protein is held in place by hydrogen bonding. Proteins are much more complex than carbohydrates or fats because of their secondary and tertiary structures and the many catalytic, regulatory and structural properties they possess.

Fats

Dietary sources of fats include meat, poultry, fish, eggs, cheese, butter, vegetable oils, nuts, and avocados. Fats are also found in smaller amounts in grains and green leafy vegetables. Like carbohydrates, fats contain hydrogen, oxygen and carbon. In this case, the building blocks are fatty acids instead of sugars.

Fats comprise a significant part of a normal diet. Consuming adequate amounts of healthy fats is critical for maintaining good health. Fats provide an excellent energy source, but also serve as building blocks for cell membranes, hormones and other fatty acid-based molecules like eicosanoids.

Hormones and eicosanoids act as messengers in the body helping to regulate a variety of processes including immunity (the ability to fight off disease). There are four different kinds of fats; monounsaturated fats, polyunsaturated fats, saturated fats and hydrogenated or trans-fats[1].

Monounsaturated fats, like those in nuts, peanut oil, olive oil and canola oil, are believed to have significant health benefits because they lower bad cholesterol (LDL) and increase good cholesterol (HDL). Meats contain both saturated and monounsaturated fats as does butter.

[1] Unsaturated fats have at least one double bond between the carbon molecules (and hence have one less hydrogen molecule attached to the carbon atom). If there is only one double bond, the fat is called monounsaturated. If there is more than one double bond the fat is called polyunsaturated. Saturated fats have no double bonds because hydrogen is bound to as many spots as are available on each carbon atom. Trans-fats are produced by a process called hydrogenation. Hydrogenation is a chemical process to add more hydrogen to natural unsaturated fats to decrease the number of double bonds. Trans-fats are considered to be unhealthy but are used because they are more resistant to oxidation (becoming rancid).

Polyunsaturated fats are found in fish as well as canola, safflower and flaxseed oil. Polyunsaturated fats tend to lower cholesterol. However, both good and bad cholesterol levels are lowered.

Saturated fats are found in a number of foods including butter, cream, coconut oil, palm oil, poultry and meats. Saturated fats have been associated with an increase in both good (HDL) and bad (LDL) cholesterol. There is a growing consensus that a certain amount of saturated fats may actually be healthy for our bodies and our immune system and should be consumed along with polyunsaturated fats.

Some fatty acids are considered non-essential because our bodies can synthesis them. But unlike amino acids, where ten are essential, there are only two essential fatty acids, the polyunsaturated omega -3 and omega-6 fatty acids. Omega-6 fatty acids are relatively prevalent in most diets due to consumption of meats from animals that were fed grains high in omega-6 fatty acids, while omega-3 fatty acids are less abundant. Good sources of omega-3 fatty acids include fish and fish oil as well as certain vegetable- based cooking oils. Beneficial effects of omega-3 fatty acids on cardiovascular disease have been reported (1).

Trans-fats generally do not occur naturally and are made by the hydrogenation of vegetable oil. This process is used to improve the shelf life of vegetable oils. Trans-fats are the unhealthiest fat and have been linked to an increase in cholesterol as well as cardiovascular disease (2, 3). The problem is that these types of oils are used in many processed foods including snack foods, peanut butter and are difficult to avoid.

Two good references for choosing healthy fats are Atkins for Life by Robert Atkins and The Low-Carb Comfort Food Cookbook by Dr. Michael and Mary Dan Eades and Ursula Solom.

Vitamins, Minerals and Water

In addition to carbohydrates, proteins and fats our bodies need water, minerals and vitamins. Vitamins aid in a variety of cellular processes and are needed to produce a number of co-enzymes that are essential for numerous metabolic activities. Most vitamins are contained in our diets but some, like vitamin K, are synthesized by bacteria in our intestines. Minerals include calcium, phosphorus and iron as well as many trace minerals. These are normally received in our diet, however, imbalances in pH or intestinal surgery can impact the effective absorption of minerals, particularly calcium and iron.

Water, though not energy yielding, is the most important single metabolic requirement we have. Water is required for the breakdown and metabolism of every food group. In addition, water is important in maintaining body temperature, osmotic balance (controlling salt and other electrolyte concentrations) and blood pressure.

The Digestive Process

Note: I have reproduced Figure 1 for this discussion.

When we eat food our teeth grind up the food breaking it into smaller pieces making it more accessible to digestive enzymes and stomach acid. Before the food leaves our mouth, digestion of carbohydrates has already begun. The saliva, produced by six salivary glands, not only acts to lubricate the food, but also contains the enzyme amylase. Amylase immediately begins breaking bonds between the sugar molecules in starches and other complex carbohydrates. This process last only until the food reaches the stomach. When we swallow, the food is pushed down the esophagus aided by the peristaltic (wave-like) action of muscles in the esophagus and by lubricating mucus also produced by cells lining the surface of the esophagus. To enter the stomach the food must pass the lower esophageal sphincter (LES). As I mentioned in chapter 2, the LES is formed by rings of muscles between the lower esophagus and the stomach. When the muscles are contracted, the sphincter is closed. When muscles relax, the sphincter is open. When food approaches the LES the muscles relax and food is able to enter the stomach. Note: The lower esophageal sphincter plays a key role determining how susceptible we are to heartburn, as you will see in chapter 5.

Stomach

By the time food arrives in the stomach, parietal cells lining the stomach have already been stimulated by histamine (in response to the smell, thought or taste of food) to produce acid. The parietal cells are capable of producing so much acid that the pH (acidity) of the stomach can be as low as 1

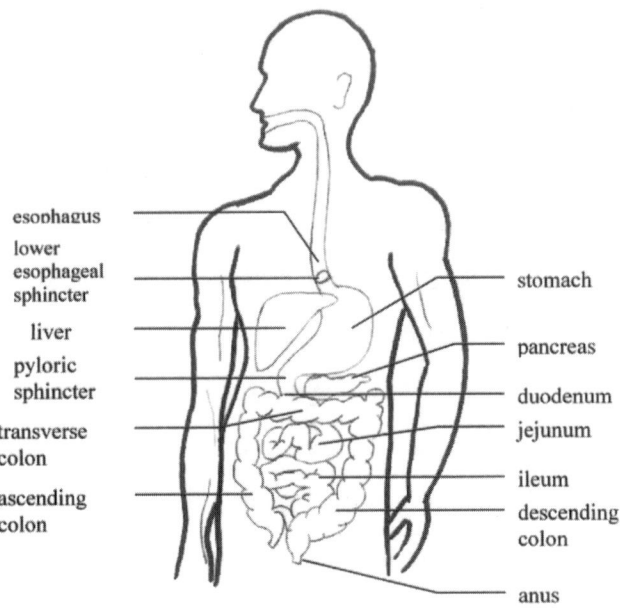

Figure 1. Human digestive system

pH unit. This pH is low enough to dissolve metal and kill bacteria. The pH scale goes from 1 to 14: 1 is extremely acidic, 14 is extremely basic, and pH 7 is considered neutral. Both extremes are very corrosive. The stomach protects itself from its own acid by secreting a thick mucus layer. Upon entering the stomach, amylase, previously produced in the saliva, is destroyed by the acid, which takes over the digestion process. The breakdown of carbohydrates (sugars including disaccharides and polysaccharides and more complex carbohydrates called starches) temporarily ceases in the stomach. Muscles contained in the stomach walls help mix the food with the acid and digestion of proteins begins. The main purpose of the stomach is the breakdown of protein although some fat is also broken down via stomach acid as well. The acid denatures (unfolds) the proteins while pepsin (the active form of pepsinogen) is released into the food-acid mixture called chyme. Pepsin, active only at very low pH, digests the large protein molecules into smaller pieces (polypeptides). After several hours of digestion, the chyme consists of a mixture of polypeptides, polysaccharides and triglycerides that represent the partial breakdown of protein, carbohydrates and fats respectively. This mixture is transferred through the pyloric sphincter (the sphincter at the distal or far end of the stomach) into the duodenum (the beginning of the small intestine).

Small Intestine

The small intestine is approximately 20 feet long. Most of this length is approximately divided between the duodenum and jejunum with only a couple of feet of length comprising the ileum. The role of the small intestine is to complete the digestive process and absorb the released nutrients into the blood.

Duodenum

In the duodenum, the first portion of the small intestine, the acid produced by the stomach is neutralized by bicarbonate produced from the pancreas and further enzymatic digestion of the mixture of polypeptides, polysaccharides and triglycerides takes place. The pancreas and gland cells of the small intestine secrete digestive enzymes such as amylase maltase, sucrase and lactase to continue the break down of polysaccharides (carbohydrates) into monosaccharides. Lipase is produced to break down fat into fatty acids. To aid in fat digestion and absorption, bile produced in the liver and stored in the gall bladder is released into the mix. Bile is like a detergent and helps emulsify (break into smaller more soluble pieces) the fat. Trypsin and chymotrypsin are produced to further break down polypeptides to amino acids. The job of the duodenum is to break down each type of food into its most basic form; fat to fatty acids, protein to amino acids and complex carbohydrates into monosaccharides. The chyme is now ready to be absorbed.

Jejunum

Most nutrient absorption occurs in the second portion of the small intestine called the jejunum. The inside surface of the jejunum is covered with finger-like projections called villi. These projections are the location of cells that contain even smaller projections called microvilli, which together form what is known as the brush boarder. The structure of the jejunum and the cellular morphology of the cells lining the jejunum create a huge amount of surface area to allow for optimal absorption of nutrients (monosaccharides, fatty acids and amino acids). The absorption process effectively passes the nutrients from protein and carbohydrate digestion through the intestinal wall into the blood via the portal vein. The nutrients from fats (fatty acids) enter intestinal epithelial cells and are transported to lacteal villi, then into lymphatics vessels and then to venous blood.

The nutrients absorbed into the blood then pass through the liver which filters out the nutrients and processes them in such a way as to remove toxins, and distribute the energy bearing molecules to the rest of the body in a tightly controlled fashion.

Ileum

Any unabsorbed food goes on to the third portion of the small intestine called the ileum where water, some vitamins and bile salts (initially used to emulsify fat) are absorbed. Water and bile salts are recycled. At this point the digestion of food and the absorption nutrients is generally considered complete although our body has one more mechanism to recover energy from food that our bodies cannot break down. Microorganisms play a role in this process, as you will see below. Approximately four to six hours after a meal the chyme leaves the small intestine via the ileocecal valve and enters the large intestine.

Large Intestine (Colon)

The large intestine is comprised of the cecum, ascending colon, transverse colon, descending colon and finally the sigmoid colon. The first part of the large intestine is called the cecum to which the appendix is connected. The liquid leaving the small intestine has been depleted of many of its nutrients as it enters the colon. What remains is a mixture of water and undigestible fiber such as cellulose. As the undigested food is pushed through the colon much of the water and electrolytes such as sodium are removed and recycled. Microorganisms present in large numbers are able to further breakdown the food that we cannot. These microbes facilitate the digestive process by producing essential amino acids, vitamins such as vitamin K and B vitamins as well as short chain fatty acids (SCFAs) including acetate, propionate and butyrate. These microbially derived products provide essential nutrients that our bodies cannot make. The absorption of SCFAs provides a means of capturing otherwise lost energy from our food. Acetate propionate and butyrate are metabolized by epithelium cells lining the large intestine (butyrate), liver cells (propionate) and muscle (acetate). The same populations of microbes also produce less desirable end products including gas (refer to chapter 5). One other role of gut microbes is the metabolism of bile acids. After the fecal matter has been sufficiently processed and dehydrated it is stored and eventually expelled via the anus. The entire digestive process takes approximately one to two days.

References:

1. Kris-Etherton PM, Harris WS, Appel LJ. Consumption, Fish Oil, Omega-3 Fatty Acids, and Cardiovascular Disease. Circulation. 2002; 106:2747.
2. Booyens J, Louwrens CC, Katzeff IE. The role of unnatural dietary trans and cis unsaturated fatty acids in the epidemiology of coronary artery disease. Med Hypotheses 1988; 25:175-182.
3. Grundy SM, Abate N, Chandalia M. Diet composition and the metabolic syndrome: what is the optimal fat intake? Am J Med. 2002 Dec 30; 113 Suppl 9B:25S-29S.

Chapter 5

A New Theory

"The Body Never Lies"
Martha Graham

In this chapter I discuss the details of my theory. I will provide evidence that GERD is caused by consuming excess carbs that our own microorganisms turn into gas. The gas pressure overwhelms weakened lower esophageal sphincter muscles in GERD patients resulting in acid reflux.

In the first chapter I discussed my own experiences treating my GERD successfully with low carb dieting. I cited the experiences of doctors including Drs. Michael and Mary Dan Eades and Dr. Atkins himself using the low carb approach to treat GERD patients. I also cited a clinical study reporting that reducing dietary carbohydrates can eliminate acid reflux and heartburn. I personally can feel a dramatic change in my digestive system after reducing my intake of carbs. I have significantly less intestinal gas, particularly in my upper digestive system, acid reflux and heartburn are gone and I no longer feel bloated. Martha Graham is right when she says, "the body never lies." The question that I have been pursuing in the last year is not "does it work?" I know it works. My question is how does it work? That is what this chapter is all about.

Refer to the working theory I proposed in the first chapter of this book:

> "Excess dietary carbohydrates escape absorption by our intestines. Microbes breakdown these carbohydrates quickly producing gas and acid as end products. The resulting gas creates intestinal pressure, which is the driving force for acid reflux. Gas is not produced in any significant amounts by the microbial breakdown of fats and proteins and therefore consumption of excess carbohydrates, but not proteins and fats, will result in heartburn in susceptible individuals."

Put more simply:

Carbohydrates + Microbes = Intestinal Gas
Intestinal Gas + Weak LES = Acid Reflux

Current Thinking on Acid Reflux

As discussed in Chapter 2, the leading theory on the cause of acid reflux is that the lower esophageal sphincter (LES) muscles (that normally provide a barrier between your stomach and esophagus) are weaker in GERD patients and that these muscles "relax" spontaneously and frequently in GERD patients allowing the sphincter to open and stomach contents to escape into the esophagus (1).

I believe the first part of this reasoning to be correct. People with GERD have weaker LES muscles. But why would the LES "relax" frequently when you are not swallowing? According to my theory, what appears as LES relaxation is actually weak LES muscles giving way to pressure (caused by gas) that builds up in the stomach. Acid reflux occurs when the gas pressure causes gastric distension (stomach bloating) that pushes the stomach contents including acid through your LES into your esophagus. This idea is supported by a study showing that in GERD patients, reflux was associated with an increase in intra-abdominal pressure (2). Also belching and heartburn in GERD patients are correlated with episodes of pathological acid reflux. (3).

Got Gas?

But where is the pressure coming from? I believe this "back pressure" builds up from the production of hydrogen (H_2), carbon dioxide (CO_2) and, in some cases methane (CH_4), by microbes in our intestinal tract feeding on excess carbohydrates. I believe that microbially produced gas is the cause of most acid reflux. If this were true, one should be able to inhibit acid reflux by either inhibiting the microbes or taking away the carbs. It turns out, that this is indeed what happens. I have already provided examples of how carb reduction can dramatically eliminate acid reflux. Taking away the carbs does work. What I learned researching this book was that administration of the antibiotic erythromycin decreases gastroesophageal reflux (4) and increases LES pressure (5). The authors interpreted these results as prokinetic (stimulate smooth muscle contraction and hence peristalsis) or motilin-like (induces stomach / intestinal contractions similar to that induced by motilin, a protein hormone) effects respectively. I believe these results can be better explained as a direct result of erythromycin's inhibitory effect on gut microorganisms.

As the microbes are inhibited by erythromycin, they will not be able to metabolize the carbs and produce gas. LES pressure (as measured for the experiment in reference 5) is increased because there is less gas pressure in the stomach to "push" on the LES forcing it open in the case of reflux. The result is decreased acid reflux. This does not mean I recommend antibiotics to treat acid reflux. Eventually erythromycin-resistant microbes would predominate, restoring gas production and in some cases causing other deleterious effects as antibiotics can upset the natural microbial balance of our intestines allowing the "unfriendly" microbes to predominate.

If gas pressure were the cause of reflux, you would expect pressure to build up if you could keep the LES closed. This is actually what happens. In the chapter on GERD treatments, I noted that anti-reflux surgery was associated with a large amount of stomach and intestinal gas. The phenomenon is referred to as "Gas-bloat syndrome." Anti-reflux surgery creates a one-way valve between the esophagus and stomach, which can result in the inability to belch and vomit. However, because patients have not been instructed to reduce their intake of carbohydrates, gas and pressure can build up. That could explain another side effect of this surgery: flatulence. The gas is trying to escape from both ends of the digestive tract. Which direction it goes depends on a number of factors, but the most significant factor may be where the gas is produced in the intestine.

Microbial Populations in the Human Gastrointestinal Tract

The intestinal tract of humans is teaming with microorganisms. Most of these microorganisms are "friendly" and play several essential roles in human digestion. We have what you might call a "mutual arrangement." We need microbes to help with digestion provide certain essential nutrients like vitamins that our bodies cannot produce. Microorganisms need to share some of our food to survive. Estimates on the total number or microbes in our body run as high as 100 to 1000 trillion, or more than our own number of human cells (6, 7). Most of the human gut microbes are bacteria although fungi, protozoa and viruses are present as well. Overall the number of species of microbes in our GI tract is estimated at greater than 400. The organisms in our gut must survive almost entirely in the absence of oxygen (the human intestine is anaerobic) and hence are capable of fermentation (gaining energy from the breakdown of nutrients in the absence of oxygen). Some bacteria identified in the human gastrointestinal (GI) tract include *Bacteroides vulgatus, Bacteroides fragilis, Bifidobacterium* sp., *Clostridium perfringens, Enterococcus faecalis, Escherichia coli, Eubacterium* sp.*, Lactobacillus* sp., and *Streptococcus* sp. During my postdoctoral studies at Tufts University in Boston Massachusetts, I studied and published on two of these organisms, *B. fragilis* and *E. coli*. I can tell you from growing them, they thrive on carbohydrates and they produce a lot of gas. *Bacteroides* species in particular are well known for being able to break down a wide variety of carbohydrates.

Where are The Microorganisms?

The stomach of healthy people is generally devoid of microorganisms because of the presence of stomach acid. (The bacterium *H. pylori* is one exception[1]).

> 1. The bacterium *H. pylori* is able to colonize the stomach in many individuals because this bacterium has evolved various means to modulate stomach acid. Because of this ability to lower stomach acid, some strains of *H. pylori* may actually play a preventative role in GERD. Unfortunately, the same organism can cause stomach and duodenal ulcers.

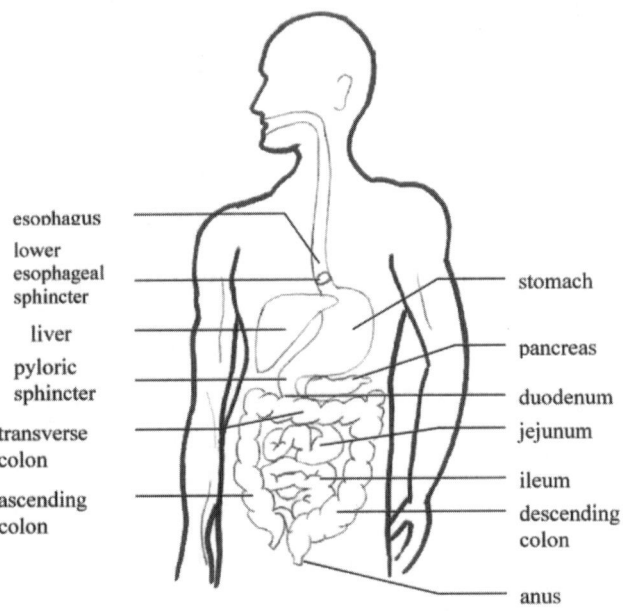

Figure1. Human digestive system

The duodenum and jejunum, towards the proximal or early part of the small intestine (closer to the stomach), reportedly have a relatively low number of resident microorganisms. The numbers range from ten thousand to one million bacteria per milliliter (mL) of intestinal contents. The distal end of the small intestine, the ileum, reportedly has more microorganisms present in the range of 10 million to 100 million bacteria per mL of the intestinal contents. The colon, or large intestine, is the primary location of most of our resident microorganisms with approximately 10 billion to 100 billion bacteria per mL (6, 8).

The Role of Microorganisms in Digestion

Microorganisms metabolize residual fiber, indigestible or unabsorbed carbohydrates, as well as some proteins, and, fats that escape absorption in the small intestine. Most microbial activity is thought to occur in the colon where most of the microorganisms reside although there is clearly microbial activity in the small intestine as well. Though microbes are able to metabolize carbohydrates, proteins and even fats, they prefer carbohydrates, particularly glucose (like our own cells) which can be most rapidly used. Carbohydrates are particularly preferred in the human gut environment that is devoid of oxygen (anaerobic). Microorganisms living in both the large intestine and in the lower small intestine are able to survive by consuming a portion of our meals using a process called fermentation. The large intestine was at one time thought to function strictly in water absorption not nutrient absorption. In fact, a significant amount of short chain fatty acids (like acetate, lactate, propionate and butyrate) produced by microbes (that ferment unabsorbed carbohydrates) are absorbed by our bodies via the large intestine (colon). That is one way we recapture energy lost when carbohydrates are not absorbed in the small intestine.

What's Happening in the Jejunum

Most intestinal absorption of fully digested protein, fats and carbohydrates occurs in the jejunum portion of the small intestine. In this region of the intestine, there is likely competition between the microbes and our own nutrient absorption system (that's why animals grow bigger when raised on feed containing antibiotics). Most of the food we consume is broken down and ready for absorption when it reaches the jejunum. Absorption by the jejunum is generally very efficient; however, not all food is absorbed. The term used is "malabsorption". Malabsorption of food has two basic causes. The first cause is the inability to breakdown food sufficiently to allow absorption. This can happen when certain individuals do not have the right enzymes to breakdown certain substances like lactose for people who are lactose intolerant. Other substances, like fiber, cannot be broken down by anyone, as people do not have enzymes capable of digesting fiber. The second cause of malabsorption is simply volume. As efficient as our digestive system is, some of the food we eat will not be absorbed simply because we are consuming more than our system is able to absorb. Food that escapes absorption in the jejunum is readily available for consumption by intestinal microbes.

Do Proteins and Fats Cause Gas?

Fats produce little, if any, gas in the intestine due to the way they are metabolized by gut microbes. Fats and oils are lipids composed of tri- and diglycerides. Bacteria secrete enzymes called lipases that break down (hydrolyze) tri- and diglycerides to free fatty acids and glycerol. Glycerol can be fermented but the fatty acids, which make up the bulk of the energy in fats, are not processed efficiently in the absence of oxygen. Because of how fats are metabolized by bacteria in our intestines (without oxygen), there is little or no gas produced and hence it makes sense that fats don't contribute to heartburn. There is growing evidence to support this rational (9, 10, 11).

The process of microbial degradation of protein in the absence of oxygen is called putrefaction. Proteins that are not completely broken down to amino acids by the time they reach the jejunum are subjected to decomposition by microbially produced enzymes. This is a relatively slow process. The proteins are broken down extracellularly and then the microorganisms only take up and further process the specific amino acids they require. As amino acids contain nitrogen the microbial breakdown products are amines and ammonia. As shown in Figure 2, amines and ammonia have a similar structure and are both basic. In fact, the pH of ammonia is eleven. For this reasons the large intestine (where most of the microbial degradation of proteins occurs) has a higher pH than the small intestine. Because proteins are broken down more slowly and the amino acids used selectively by gut microbes, less gas is produced and it is produced in the more distal regions of large intestine (further from the stomach). Any gas produced from proteins is likely to contribute more to flatus gas than to heartburn. Also, the end products of protein breakdown are basic (as opposed to acidic). The diagram below shows how amines produced from protein breakdown are similar to ammonia and hence also have a high pH (the opposite of acid). The fact that carbohydrates result in acid production while proteins result in base production may also have an impact on heartburn, although this remains to be confirmed.

A New Theory

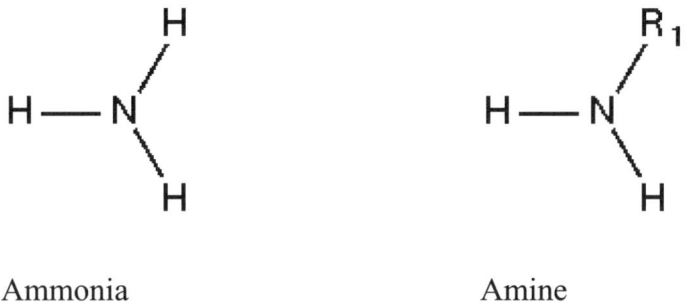

Ammonia   Amine

Figure 2. Products of protein breakdown

Microbial Breakdown of Carbohydrates

If little gas is produced from proteins and fats, that leaves carbohydrates. Carbohydrates that are not absorbed in the small intestine are rapidly consumed by microorganisms. As microbes metabolize carbohydrates, they rapidly produce significant amounts of acid and gas earlier in the digestive track, closer to the stomach. The gas pressure drives acid reflux. The acidic end products include lactic acid, acetic acid, propionic acid and butyric acid, which significantly lower the pH in the region of the intestine where they are produced. Gases produced include carbon dioxide (CO_2), hydrogen (H_2) and (in some cases) methane (CH_4).

As noted previously, carbohydrates include fiber, which cannot be digested or absorbed, as well as simple sugars and starches that are digested and absorbed by our intestines. Consumed in moderation, starches are broken down to simple sugars, like glucose, which are rapidly absorbed into the bloodstream from the small intestine. Nothing is left over for the microorganisms. However, if starches and simple sugars are consumed in excess, more of these carbs will escape absorption and become available for the intestinal microbes to metabolize resulting in intestinal gas. Essentially all of the fiber we consume (approximately 12 grams / day) escapes absorption while between 15 and 20 % of the starch we consume (approximately 30 to 40 grams per day) has been estimated to escape absorption (12, 13). It is known with certainty that a significant amount of gas is produced by bacteria in our intestines in response to carbohydrate metabolism. In fact, there have been explosions during intestinal surgery due to high amounts of hydrogen and methane gas production (14, 15, 16). Carbon dioxide formed in the gut by gut microbes and by our own digestive process, as stomach acid is neutralized by bicarbonate in the duodenum, is less of a problem because this gas is absorbed more efficiently by our intestines. I believe hydrogen, and in some cases methane (not everyone produces methane), are the real culprits.

According to Suarez and Levitt (17), 30 g of carbohydrate that escapes absorption in a day could produce more than 10,000 mL (ten liters) of hydrogen gas. That is a huge amount of gas! As hydrogen is being formed by some types of bacteria, however, it is also being used by other bacteria for methane production or sulfate reduction (18). The point is that during this metabolic balancing act between the microbes in our intestines there is a lot of gas being produced. I believe microbially produced gas resulting from excess carbohydrate consumption is the main cause of heartburn in susceptible individuals. If these susceptible individuals (that have weaker sphincter muscles) reduce the amount of carbohydrates they consume, it makes sense that they will produce much less gas and their reflux symptoms will subside. This is, in fact what happens.

The amount of excess carbohydrate consumed, the complexity of the carbohydrates, as well as the type of carbohydrate (how the sugars are linked together) will determine the intensity of the microbial activity, the amount of gas and acid that is produced, and even the intestinal location where gas and acid are produced.

Gas and Acid Reflux

The problem (reflux) arises when excess gas production in the small intestine and proximal or early part of the large intestine overwhelms the normal means for its removal. Excess gas that is not absorbed into the blood, vented through the anus via flatus or metabolized by other microorganisms in the intestine will exert pressure. The pressure pushes intestinal contents from the duodenum back into the stomach via the pyloric sphincter. As the gas (and intestinal contents) enters the stomach, it creates pressure inside the stomach. In susceptible individuals, the gas pressure results in gastroesophageal reflux. If you have a relatively weak lower esophageal sphincter, you will likely have heartburn in response to a high carb diet. From an evolutionary standpoint, weaker lower esophageal sphincters were not a disadvantage because thousands of years ago our diets were significantly lower in carbohydrates. It is the excess carbohydrates in the USDA Food Pyramid that pushes GERD sufferer's lower esophageal sphincters beyond their limit.

How could gas from the intestine get into the stomach?

The pyloric sphincter is positioned at the bottom of the stomach separating it from the duodenum. Duodenal reflux (reflux of partially digested food back into the stomach from the duodenum) occurs when partially digested food is refluxed back into the stomach past the pyloric sphincter. Duodenal reflux coupled with lower esophageal sphincter reflux is one of four natural mechanisms to allow excess gas (the product of microbial carbohydrate metabolism) to escape from the intestine, the other three being absorption of gas into the blood stream, flatus (farting) and metabolism of the gases by other microorganisms inhabiting the gut. With enough gas pressure, duodenal contents can flow backwards into the stomach.

Duodenal Reflux and GERD

There is growing evidence that duodenal contents are at work in GERD. According to Dr. James Christensen (19), "Other elements besides the hydrogen ions in the gastric content contribute to the damage that the gastric juice inflicts on the squamous epithelium of the esophagus. Enzymes and bile salts in the gastric juice clearly augment the damaging effects of the acid. Bile often gets into the gastric content because of duodenogastric reflux. Both the sphincteric function of the pylorus and of duodenal peristalsis act to oppose such reflux, but they often fail to do this well enough, allowing enough bile to flow back into the stomach to produce inflammation of the epithelium in the gastric antrum. Such antral gastritis very often accompanies GERD because the bile-contaminated gastric juice also enters the esophagus in gastroesophageal reflux".

Sequence of Events (refer to figures 3 and 4)

To better understand the susceptibility of GERD patients to carbohydrates, let's look at three scenarios with visual diagrams to relate to.

1. Someone susceptible to heartburn consumes a meal low in carbohydrates: As shown in figure 3, the food is digested and most of the carbohydrates present are absorbed in the small intestine. Some will not be absorbed and microbes are competing for their share. Yet there are very few carbohydrates available and hence the microbes produce only a small amount of gas in the upper intestine. Hence there is little gas

pressure and the intestinal contents and gas are not forced back into the stomach. That means that gas pressure in the stomach is low and there is not sufficient force to drive acid reflux.

2. The same person (susceptible to heartburn) consumes a meal high in carbohydrates: As shown in figure 4, the food is digested and many of the carbs are absorbed in the small intestine (our digestion and absorption apparatus is very efficient). In this scenario, however, a significant portion or the carbohydrates escape digestion and / or absorption. As the microbes compete for this preferred energy source, much gas and acid is produced and produced closer to the duodenum and stomach. The gas produced causes pressure on the small intestine. The gas pressure literally pushes undigested food, along with much of the gas, back into the stomach creating pressure in the stomach and forcing food, acid and duodenal contents into the esophagus. The weakened lower esophageal sphincter yields to the gas pressure.

3. Someone without GERD consumes a high carbohydrate meal: Even though scenario two is initiated, this person possesses stronger lower

esophageal sphincter muscles and gas and pressure produced by microbes from excess carbs is not able to push past the LES. So people with strong lower esophageal sphincter muscles can consume significantly higher levels of carbohydrates and still not get heartburn.

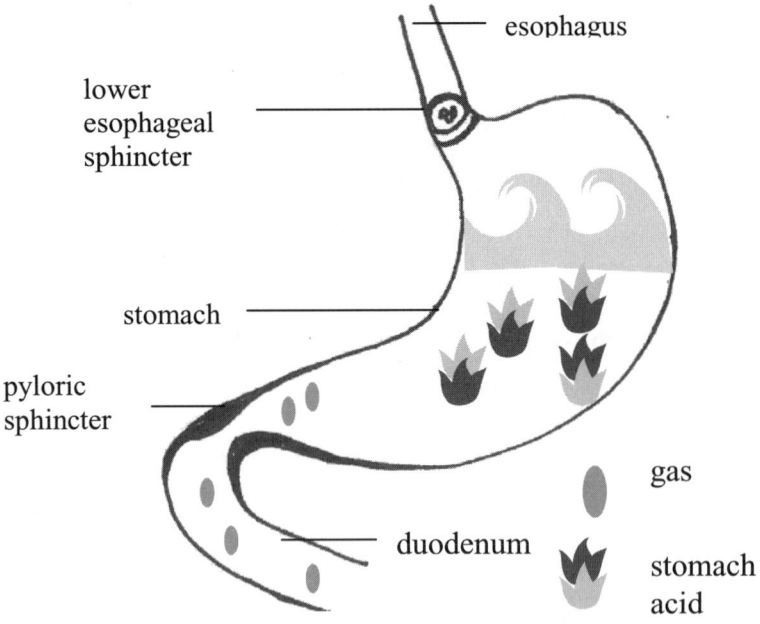

Figure 3. Digestion without excess carbohydrates

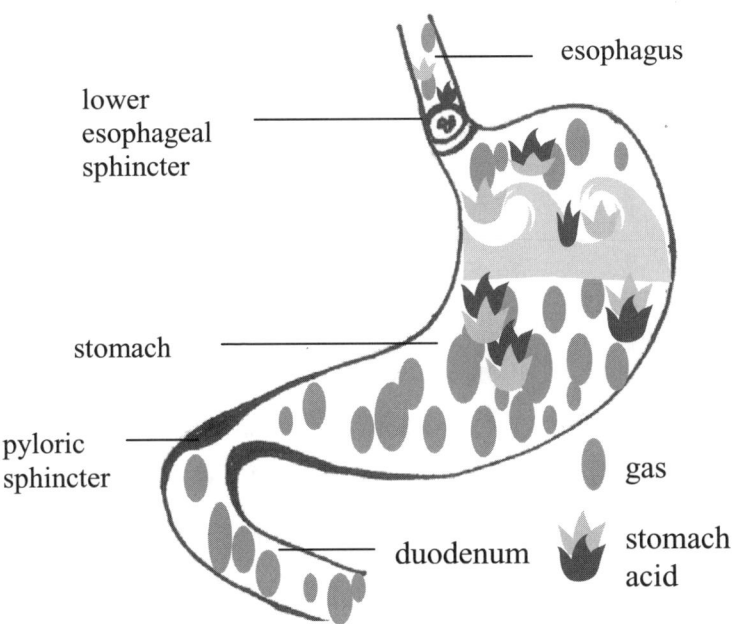

Figure 4. Excess carbohydrates result in gas pressure that drives reflux

Malabsorption

Certain carbohydrates such as lactulose are not broken down or absorbed by our intestinal track. For example, when lactulose is ingested, no breakdown or absorption takes place in our bodies, but microorganisms can metabolize lactulose, and so produce acid and gas. Hydrogen produced from the fermentation of lactulose can be detected in a breath test because some of the hydrogen produced is absorbed into the blood and exhaled via the lungs. Since human metabolism does not produce any hydrogen, the hydrogen detected must arise from the microbial breakdown of the lactulose.

Consistent with my hypothesis is the finding that intestinal fermentation of indigestible carbohydrates by microbes increases the rate of TLESRs (transient lower esophageal sphincter relations), the number of acid reflux episodes, and the symptoms of GERD (20). The indigestible carbohydrate used in the study was fructooligosaccharide (FOS), which is known to produce intestinal gas (21).

The consumption of excess carbs results in a phenomenon similar to carbohydrate malabsorption. That is, intestinal absorption of carbs can be limited by the sheer volume of carbs. The unabsorbed carbs are rapidly metabolized my microorganisms producing acid and gas resulting in heartburn. Figure 5 shows the cycle of excess carbohydrate consumption and acid reflux.

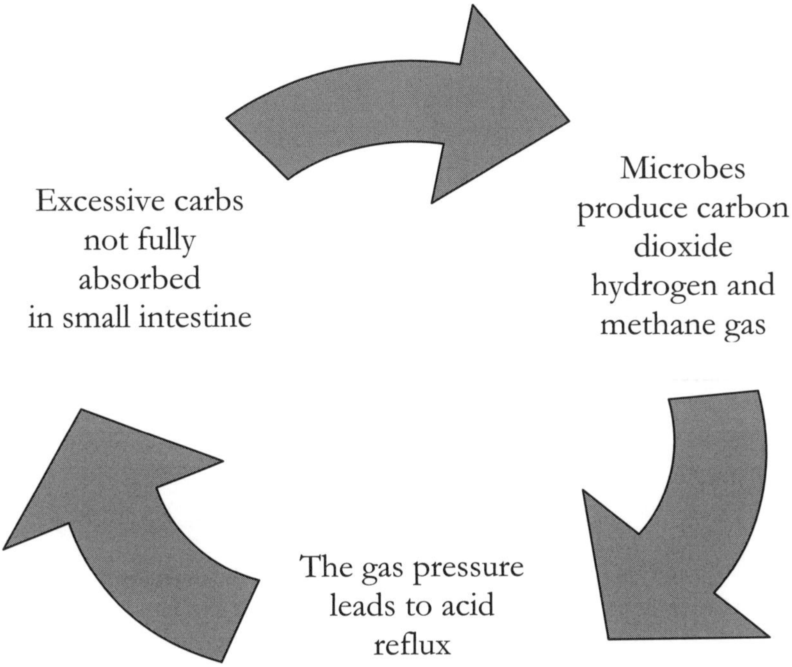

A New Theory

Excessive carbs not fully absorbed in small intestine → Microbes produce carbon dioxide hydrogen and methane gas → The gas pressure leads to acid reflux →

Figure 5. Excess consumption of carbohydrates leads to a cycle of gas pressure and acid reflux.

Carbonated Soft Drinks

I became interested in a recent study led by Mohandas Mallath at Tata Memorial Hospital in India presented at the Digestive Disease Week conference in New Orleans Louisiana in May 2004, that found a strong correlation between the rise in per capita consumption of carbonated soft drinks in the past 20 years and the increasing rates of esophageal cancer in the United States. According to the study, consumption of carbonated soft drinks rose by more than 450 percent, from 10.8 gallons per person per year in 1946 to 49.2 gallons per person per year in 2000. At the same time, during the last 25 years, rates of esophageal cancer have increased more than 570 percent among American white males.

While all studies of this nature (that make a correlation but do not show causality) need to be followed up with well controlled clinical trials, the study proposes that there is a biological basis to explain the increased duration of esophageal exposure to acid as the consumption of carbonated soft drinks increases. The rational proposed is that carbonated soft drinks are related to gastric distension, which can trigger reflux. I find this concept fascinating because it makes sense that carbonated beverages will cause stomach distention as CO_2 gas is released in the stomach. According to Mallath, "If you drink a quarter of a liter of water, your stomach distends by a quarter of a liter, but if it's a carbonated drink, your stomach may distend to maybe half a liter". This causes reflux - the acid of the stomach is thrown back into the food pipe." I give this team credit for finding this correlation, but don't believe they fully understood the basis for their conclusions.

My theory clearly assigns microbially produced gas (not only the CO_2 gas from carbonated beverages in the stomach) as the main cause of acid reflux. My own heartburn disappeared after I reduced my intake of carbohydrates, yet I continued consuming carbonated beverages at the same rate, both before and after reducing my carb intake. The only difference is that I always drank diet soda (no sugar) exclusively, both before and after starting low carb dieting. This suggests to me that the carbonation in soft drinks is not the cause of acid reflux. Currently, on my reduced carb diet, I still belch after a diet soda, but the heartburn is gone. Interestingly, most carbonated beverages are loaded with the worst form of carbohydrate, simple sugars. I believe it is the intestinal gas produced by microorganisms feeding on the sugar in most carbonated beverages that drives acid reflux by pushing duodenal contents and stomach contents past the lower esophageal sphincter into the esophagus

If the sugar in carbonated beverages is the culprit and responsible for the (reflux-mediated) rise in esophageal cancer, then one would expect the same level of risk consuming any foods containing excess sugars. That means drinking milk (containing lactose) or fruit juice (containing fructose) could also put people at risk for esophageal cancer. According to my theory there is a connection between acid reflux and consuming excess carbohydrates in general. It follows that reducing carbohydrates in general may help prevent esophageal cancer.

Complex vs. Simple Carbohydrates - Glycemic Index

Simple Carbs

There is a balance between the complexity of the carbohydrate and how quickly and efficiently it is absorbed. This is referred to as the glycemic index. Rapidly metabolizable carbohydrates (simple starches and mono and disaccharides) have a high glycemic index meaning they have a better chance of being absorbed rapidly and hence will be less available for microbial consumption. You might conclude from this rational that foods with a high glycemic index will not cause heartburn because they are absorbed so quickly. However, if large amounts of these simple carbohydrates are consumed, some will escape absorption by our bodies. These carbohydrates will be rapidly metabolized sooner by microbes due to their less complex structure. Increases in consumption of simple carbohydrates like refined sugar have been shown to result in an increase in microbial gas production in the intestines (22). In a separate study with infants being evaluated for gastroesophageal reflux (GER), increases in the concentration of glucose (dextrose) solutions produced significantly more GER (23). The lesson is that simple sugars can cause intestinal gas and GER. That is why people complain about heartburn symptoms from milk, sugar, candy and chocolate. All of these foods contain simple sugars.

Complex Carbs

Complex carbohydrates are broken down more slowly and hence have a lower glycemic index. This is the same reason they tend to raise blood glucose (and hence insulin) more slowly. Because complex carbohydrates possess a structure that is highly cross-linked, they take longer to breakdown and hence are less available for both absorption and microbial degradation as early in the digestive process. By the time complex carbohydrates with low glycemic indices are broken down to monosaccharides many of them may have already passed the small intestine (where most nutrient absorption takes place) and are entering the colon, or large intestine. When the microbes finally are able to utilize complex carbohydrates (now monosaccharides) gas production will be more likely to dissipate in the form of flatus gas due to its distal (far from the stomach) location in the intestinal tract. A good example is beans (low glycemic index), which tend to cause flatulence. I don't think this means that you can eat as many complex carbohydrates as you want. If you consume enough, microbes will likely metabolize enough of these excess complex carbs fast enough to contribute to earlier gas production and hence heartburn.

The take home message is that intestinal gas is the root cause of acid reflux. Intestinal gas of concern is produced primarily from microbial metabolism of excess carbohydrates, because unlike fats and proteins, carbohydrates are more readily and more rapidly utilized by microbes resulting in significant volumes of intestinal gas. Both simple and complex carbohydrates can contribute to acid reflux and heartburn in susceptible individuals.

References

1. Castell DO, Murray JA, Tutuian R, Orlando RC, Arnold R. Review article: the pathophysiology of gastro-oesophageal reflux disease - esophageal manifestations. Aliment Pharmacol Ther. 2004 Dec; 20 Suppl 9:14-25.
2. Dodds WJ, Dent J, Hogan WJ, Helm JF, Hauser R, Patel GK, Egide MS. Mechanisms of gastroesophageal reflux in patients with reflux esophagitis. N Engl J Med. 1982 Dec 16; 307(25):1547-52.
3. Lin M, Triadafilopoulos G. Belching: dyspepsia or gastroesophageal reflux disease? Am J Gastroenterol. 2003 Oct; 98(10):2139-45.
4. Pehl C, Pfeiffer A, Wendl B, Stallwag B, Kaess H. Effect of erythromycin on postprandial gastroesophageal reflux in reflux esophagitis. Dis Esophagus. 1997 Jan; 10(1):37-37.
5. Pennathur A, Tran A, Cioppi M, Fayad J, Sieren GL, Little Ag. Erythromycin strengthens the defective lower esophageal sphincter in patients with

gastroesophageal reflux disease. Am J Surg. 1994 Jan; 167(1):169-173.

6. Cummings, JH, Mcfarlene, GT, Drasar, BS. The Gut Microflora and its Significance In Gastrointestinal and Oesophageal Pathology R. Whitehead Ed. Churchill Livingstone. Edinburgh London Melbourne and New York 1989.

7. Anderson, DB. Enteritis Symposium July 9-11, 2002 Intestinal Microbes - When Does Normality Change into a Health and Performance Insult, "Abstract", B-3 to B-9.

8. Hao WL, Lee YK. Methods Mol Biol. 2004; 268:491-502.

9. Cattedra di Gastroenterologia. Fat and gastro-oesophageal reflux disease. Eur J Gastroenterol Hepatol. 2000 Dec; 12(12):1343-5.

10. Pehl, C., Waizenhoefer, A., Wendl, B., et al., "Effect of Low and High Fat Meals on Lower Esophageal Sphincter Motility and Gastroesophageal Reflux in Healthy Subjects," American Journal of Gastroenterology, 94(5), 1999, pages 1192-1196.

11. Ruhl, CE and Everhart, JE. Annals of Epidemiology. 1999: 424-435. Overweight, but Not High Dietary

Fat Intake, Increases Risk of Gastroesophageal Reflux Disease Hospitalization: The NHANES I Epidemiologic Followup Study.

12. Englyst HN, Cummings JH. Resistant starch, a "new" food component: a classification of starch for nutritional purposes. In: Morton ID ed. Cereals in a European context. Chichester: Elms Horwood, 1987: pp 221-233.

13. Bingham SA, Williams PR, Cummings J. Dietary fibre consumption in Britain: new estimates and their relation to large bowel cancer mortality. Br. J Cancer 1985; 52: 399-403.

14. Dener IA, Demirci C. Explosion during diathermy gastrotomy in a patient with carcinoma of the antrum. Int J Clin Pract. 2003 Oct; 57(8):737-8.

15. Bigard M-A, Gaucher P, Lassalle C. Fatal colonic explosion during colonoscopic polypectomy. Gastroenterology 1979; 77: 1307-1310.

16. Avgerinos A, Kalantziz N, Rekoumis G, Pallikaris G, Arapakis G, Kanaghinis T. Bowel preparation and the risk of explosion during colonoscopic polypectomy. Gut 1984; 25: 361-364.

17. Suarez F, Levitt M. Textbook of Primary and Acute Care Medicine, edited by Gideon Bosker. Part VI, Section 107.
18. Gibson GR, Cummings JH, Macfarlane GT, Allison C, Segal I, Vorster HH, Walker AR. Alternative pathways for hydrogen disposal during fermentation in the human colon. Gut 1990;31:679-683.
19. Christensen J. Division of Gastroenterology-Hepatology, Department of Internal Medicine. The University of Iowa College of Medicine, Iowa City, IA. Note: Internally reviewed statement.
20. Piche T, des Varannes SB, Sacher-Huvelin S, Holst JJ, Cuber JC, Galmiche JP. Colonic fermentation influences lower esophageal sphincter function in gastroesophageal reflux disease. Gastroenterology. 2003 Apr; 124(4):894-902.
21. Oku T, Nakamura S. Eur J Clin Nutr. 2003 Sep; 57(9):1150-6. Comparison of digestibility and breath hydrogen gas excretion of fructo-oligosaccharide, galactosyl-sucrose, and isomalto-oligosaccharide in healthy human subjects.
22. Kruis, W, Forstmaier, G, Scheurien C, Stellaard, F. Effect of diets low and high in refined sugars on gut

transit, bile acid metabolism, and bacterial fermentation. Gut. 1991. 32(4): 367-71.
23. Sutphen JL, Dillard VL. Dietary caloric density and osmolality influence gastroesohpageal reflux in infants. Gastroenterology. 1989 Sep; 97(3): 601-604.

Chapter 6

My GERD Friendly Diet

"I cannot help notice that there is no problem between us that cannot be solved by your (excess carbs) departure"
Mark Twain

Goodbye to Excess Carbs

According to my theory heartburn patients suffer as a direct result of consuming excess carbohydrates. Many of the carbohydrates escape absorption in the small intestine and, instead, are consumed by gut microorganisms. The result is the production of significant amounts of gas. The gas pressure pushes partially digested food back into the stomach and then past a weakened lower esophageal sphincter into the esophagus causing acid reflux. It makes perfect sense that the way to treat heartburn is to reduce your intake of carbohydrates. This chapter will show you how to adjust your carbohydrate intake to remove the excess fuel that your own microbes use to produce reflux-causing gas.

My diet plan uses a four-step process to gain the upper hand on heartburn. In the first step (decompression), carbs, which are fuel for gas-producing microbes, need to be significantly limited to ensure that heartburn is stopped. After stopping your heartburn, steps two and three help you gradually add back carbohydrates using your symptoms, or lack of symptoms, as a guide until you have determined your optimal level of carbohydrate intake that will allow you to remain symptom free. The last step (permanent relief) helps you develop a maintenance diet that will allow you to control heartburn on a permanent basis. To support you in curing your heartburn, I discuss each of the food groups that make up a healthy low carb diet. I have incorporated several tables at the end of the chapter listing the carb levels in numerous foods from all of the food groups. I also provide tips and advice as well as additional reading to help you embrace a low carb lifestyle specifically designed to eliminate heartburn. No one wants to have their food choices limited, but if it means eliminating heartburn and there are very enjoyable and satisfying alternatives available it makes sense to give it a try. You can do what millions of others have done. That is, to enjoy life and eating without overindulging in carbohydrates. My dietary plan is designed to help you eat a varied diet with as many food choices as possible, including carbohydrates, while remaining heartburn free.

According to Dr. Michael and Mary Dan Eades and Ursula Solom (The Low Carb Comfort Cook Book), it is estimated that as many as 25 million North Americans have followed or currently follow some variation of the low-carb nutritional theme. The biggest reason for reducing carbs has been weight loss but stopping acid reflux can now be added increasing the momentum of this incredible and healthy trend. As low carbohydrate dieting continues to gain momentum and people realize all the health benefits from eating the way our bodies evolved to eat (more protein and healthy fats and less carbohydrates) we will see more and more healthy, tasty and enjoyable alternatives to high carb foods emerge in the supermarkets. A week does not go by that I don't discover new low carb products to experiment with.

Curing Your Heartburn

In making this dietary change you will need to significantly reduce your carbohydrate intake. But it will not be as bad as you might imagine. If you have never tried this, it may seem a little scary, but don't worry, many people have done it, even before there were products such as Splenda to replace sugar in baking, drinks, and desserts. As you begin reducing your excess carbohydrate intake, you will increase the amount of protein and fat in your diet. Don't be afraid of fat (as long as you keep away from too many trans-fats, as you should do no matter what diet you're on), as fats are your new main energy source along with protein. Remember that proteins and fats produce less gas for the reasons I have explained based on their molecular make up and they way they are digested and metabolized by microorganisms in our intestines.

The Benefits My Low Carb Heartburn Diet

There are many advantages with my low carb dietary approach for treating heartburn. You don't have to pick and choose, make a list, keep a logbook or try to identify every little thing that either helps your heartburn or exacerbates it. It's not the coffee, it's not the cigarettes, it's not lying down, it's not the salt (contrary to a recent study) or drinking alcohol and it's not stress. It's the carbs! The aim of my diet plan is to control heartburn by reducing dietary intake of carbs to a level that eliminates symptoms. Your symptoms provide the perfect tool to monitor and adjust your carbohydrate intake level. After the initial week of low carb dieting to put the brakes on heartburn, you can begin increasing the amounts of carbs in your diet until you reach a level of carbohydrates that lets you enjoy some of your favorite carbs, sweets and desserts yet leaves you heartburn free. My diet also allows for what would be considered cheating by other low carb diets. That means that you can decide to eat high carb meals here and there knowing that you have an "ace in the hole" and can reduce your carb levels to stop heartburn if or when it reappears.

Net Carbs

Net carbs refer to those carbs that impact insulin levels. That is the total number of carbohydrates minus fiber and sugar alcohols. Most foods list total carbohydrates with the fiber, sugar and sugar alcohols listed separately. The fiber and sugar alcohols can be subtracted from the total carbohydrates to determine net carbs. Low carb foods generally list net carbs on the label.

Getting Started

As you begin this diet, be sure to check with your doctor to ensure that you have no underlying special medical conditions, which might make low carb dieting a poor choice for you. Be sure you understand the basics behind low carb dieting. Protein Power is a great book on the biochemistry and general health benefits of low carb dieting. I recommend taking a multivitamin and calcium supplement daily and drinking plenty of water. Now that you know a little more about how excess carbohydrates but not proteins or fats cause heartburn, let's turn to the practical side of things. What should I eat? How many grams of carbs can I consume? Is this going to be difficult?

Week 1 - Decompression (25 Grams of Net Carbs Per Day)

To begin this diet you need to significantly reduce your net carbohydrate intake overall. I call this phase decompression because you will be greatly reducing the fuel that allows your intestinal microbes to produce gas. I recommend limiting your total net carbs to 25 grams per day. Reducing your net carbs to 25 grams per day will ensure a drastic reduction in intestinal gas and resulting heartburn. Remember, the typical western diet contains approximately 250 - 350 grams of carbs per day (you will be reducing your carb intake by over 10 fold initially). At 25 grams net carbs per day, you should begin to loose any extra pounds as well.

As for your heartburn, you should feel the results within a couple of days. If you are like most heartburn sufferers, your heartburn symptoms will cease completely or at least be drastically reduced. Remember, you are in the process of changing your metabolism and that of your friends the gut microbes. As you change your diet, you will be causing a shift in the biochemical pathways used by the microbes as they adapt to the decrease in carbs and increase in proteins and fats. You will also be causing shifts in the populations of different microbes in your intestines by changing the ratio of protein, fat and carbohydrate. Some microbes will be better equipped to live off your new diet, some will not. There will be a mini evolution in your intestines. Don't worry, you will end up with a new but friendly population of microbes that will continue to aid your digestive process and help supply you with needed nutritional factors.

Week 2 - Equilibrium (45 Grams of Net Carbs Per Day)

After one week at 25 grams net carbs per day, your heartburn symptoms should be totally absent or greatly reduced and your digestive system should be reaching equilibrium in terms of gas pressure. That is, most of the carbs you consume are being fully absorbed and very little will be left over for the microbes to use to produce intestinal gas. (If you still have symptoms but appear to be improving, you may want to advance only to 30 or 35 grams net carbs per day for an additional week. Remember, your body does not actually need carbs as long as you are getting your calcium and taking a daily vitamin supplement.

If your heartburn has ceased, you can now continue increasing your intake of carbohydrates gradually. I would recommend increasing your net carbs by as much as 20 additional daily grams of net carbs (45 grams nets carbs total per day). As you increase your intake of carbs, keep in mind that you cannot return to the days of excess carbs. (Your upper limit of daily net carbs will be approximately 1/6 of what you previously consumed). Your target level for daily net carbs should be based on any return of heartburn symptoms as well as unwanted weight gain, if that is one of your concerns. Monitor your symptoms. If you begin to experience episodes of heartburn, you may be particularly sensitive to the effects of carbs and need to stay at the lower end of the net carb range (25 to 35 grams per day). Do not continue to increase you daily net carb levels unless you are symptom free at 45 grams net carbs per day.

Week 3 Testing the Waters (70 to 100 Grams of Net Carbs Per Day)

If, after completing the second phase of the diet (45 grams net carbs per day), you are completely heartburn free, you can experiment with higher net carb levels. Add more net carbs per day to find your upper limit (the highest level of daily net carbs that leave you heartburn free). Once you find your own net carb limit and comfort level, not only will your heartburn be a thing of the past, your general health will improve dramatically.

Week 4 Permanent Relief (Tailored net carb daily intake level that controls heartburn)

I personally keep my net carb levels below 60 grams per day mostly to keep my weight under control but also because I am particularly sensitive to the effects of carbs and I know that my symptoms will reappear if I go much higher. The reason for exploring higher levels is to test your digestive system and determine your own personal carbohydrate tolerance levels to control your heartburn (and weight for many of us). Being able to consume higher levels of net carbs will not make you healthier, it just allows for a more free and enjoyable dietary lifestyle if you can include more carbs in your diet. Remember it is your symptoms and your willingness to tolerate them that should guide your net carb level in your final maintenance diet.

Your sensitivity to carbs depends on your own lower esophageal sphincter muscle tension as well as the types of microbes in your intestine and the efficiency of your digestive system to breakdown and absorb carbs. Excess carbs will be consumed by your resident microbes resulting in the production of gas. If enough gas is produced, your symptoms will reappear.

Some heartburn sufferers may be able to tolerate relatively large amounts of carbs without symptoms (over 100 grams of net carbs per day) while others will not be able to remain heartburn free at the high end of range and will need to remain on lower levels of net carbs (25 to 45 grams per day). Keep in mind that you are experimenting at this point to determine just how many grams of carbs your own body can tolerate before your heartburn symptoms reappear. I believe that staying under 60 grams of net carbs per day will keep most heartburn sufferers free of symptoms, but if this does not work for you, just reduce your net carbs level until your symptoms abate.

Cheating

After being on this diet for over a year, I don't really count carbs anymore. When you are accustomed to eating low carb, you know what levels of net carbs are associated with various foods and can just go by your symptoms. Because I tend to gain weight at carb levels beyond 60 grams per day, I tend to stay under that range. Out of habit I generally do not eat potatoes, pasta, high carb breads, rice or other high carb foods, but frequently, I cheat.

By cheating I mean consciously deciding to eat high carb foods or go over my usual amount of daily carbs. Typically I cheat when I want to try certain recipes at a restaurant, have friends or family over or when I am on vacation; I may just go full on carb. Or, at a lunch meeting I may just grab one of those big chocolate chip cookies knowing full well the cookie alone has 30 grams of carbs. I may decide to eat two. It is not uncommon for me to have pizza and M&Ms with my family on a Friday night watching a movie. I know these foods have high carb levels and so does my carb conscious family. But by experimenting, I have found that I generally need to consume significantly higher levels of carbs (well over my 60 gram maintenance level) over two to three days for my heartburn to return. Eventually it does. In writing this book, I have purposefully reverted to high carb eating several times to see what happens. Within two to three days of consuming high carb meals and snacks, my heartburn reappears, although at reduced levels compared to my pre diet days.

Consequences

What do you do if your heartburn returns after cheating? Simply reduce your daily net carbs. It's really that simple. If my cheating or experimentation (call it what you will) leads to heartburn symptoms I simply revert to what has become my low carb way of eating. I am perfectly happy with soy milk on low carb cereal or eggs and bacon or low carb pancakes (and low carb syrup) for breakfast. I keep mixed nuts and other low carb goodies at my desk for snacks. For lunch I may have a chef or Greek salad, a sandwich with low carb bread or low carb wrap or, in a pinch, a bun-less cheeseburger. For dinner I am perfectly happy with a nice steak or piece of salmon with asparagus, broccoli, salad or spinach followed by low carb ice cream over a low carb brownie. Don't forget to enjoy a nice glass of wine with your dinner. Wine (dry red or white) is only 2 – 3 grams net carbs per glass.

Foods

To get an idea of the types of foods that comprise reduced carb eating this section provides examples of proteins, acceptable carbohydrates and fats.

Proteins

Proteins include foods such as seafood, meat, eggs, cheese, and poultry as well as vegetable protein like soy milk. Proteins are also plentiful in cottage cheese and sour cream. Most protein-based foods also contain needed fats. Meats like steak, hamburger, sausage, pork chops, bacon, roasts and ribs are a great place to start. To add variety, try meals using chicken, turkey, duck or seafood like salmon, tuna, bass, scallops, or shrimp. I also use pre-sliced turkey, salami, vegetables and various cheeses for my roll ups. (Note that prepared meats including bacon contain significant amounts of nitrates, which are not healthy. Try to limit these by eating fresh meats where possible.)

While on this reduced carb heartburn diet, take advantage of the opportunity to explore the many cheeses with very different tastes and properties. The Europeans have really outdone us here and have a tremendous variety of excellent cheeses from common and affordable to refined, exotic and expensive. One of my favorite cheeses is regular goat cheese. I enjoy goat cheese in salads (especially Greek Salad) and in omelets. Sharp cheddar is also one of my favorites. Pre shredded cheeses are convenient for salads, quesadillas and cooked broccoli. Another recipe I use was given to me by a colleague at work and involves Parmesan cheese. You bake (fresh) Parmesan cheese on a cookie sheet to make a snack that comes out a bit like crackers.

Carbohydrates

Carbohydrates are present in literally every plant although some plants contain more fiber (heartburn friendly) while others contain more starch and simple sugars (heartburn unfriendly). It is the high starch vegetables that contain the most net carbs. As much as possible, avoid starchy foods like potatoes, corn, flour, regular bread, regular pasta, and cereal. There are low carb almond, soy, bran and whey-based recipes for low carb baking that produce breads, pancakes, waffles, crepes, and even low carb pasta and pizza that will satisfy your carb cravings. I am currently reading Dr. Michael and Mary Dan Eades, and Ursula Solom's new book, "The Low-Carb Comfort Cook Book" that is just fantastic. Several low carb breads are now available in markets as well as my favorite, low carb tortilla wraps. I use these frequently to make breakfast burritos, lunch roll-ups and quesadillas (Refer to Dana Carpenter's 15-Minute Low-Carb Recipes for many excellent tortilla recipes). Instead of potatoes or pasta, I generally have an extra helping of low carb vegetables, a slice of avocado (great source of healthy fat as well), salad, a side of coleslaw (sweetened with Splenda), or one of the recipes mentioned above. A variety of side dishes that mimic rice can be prepared from cauliflower. Fran McCullough came up the idea in her book, Living Low Carb. Dana Carpenter in her book, 15-Minute Low-Carb Recipes, has expanded significantly on this concept providing many more tasty "rice" recipes using cauliflower.

As you begin to increase your net daily carbs, remember that high fiber / low starch vegetables can be consumed in more liberal quantities. High fiber / low carb veggies include spinach, lettuce, celery and all greens as well as broccoli, asparagus, cabbage, avocado, garlic, onions and peppers (use onions and peppers in limited amounts for flavor, since onions and peppers do have more carbs). Carrots have higher carb counts than the foods listed above, but can be grated to add color and flavor to your salads and dishes without adding many carbs. The same goes for tomatoes. While a healthy part of your diet can include tomatoes, use these at reasonable levels considering your overall carb maintenance level.

Nuts and seeds are high in protein, low in starch and very nutritious. The variety of nuts is tremendous and can be used for snacks, in dishes or on salads. Walnuts, peanuts, pecans, pistachios, brazil nuts and others are excellent alternatives to high carb shacks. I also eat a variety of seeds as a source of protein and vitamins without adding too many carbs. If you are like me, you may find nuts addictive, so consider your overall carb counts and set some limits.

Fruits are one carbohydrate food group that deserves special mention. I try to stay away from consuming apples, plums, bananas, oranges, grapes, raisins, grapefruits, and other very sweet fruits. These fruits tend to contain the higher levels of carbs. Though many fruits are reported to have lower glycemic indexes (absorbed more slowly) than grain-based foods and may be considered the healthy alternative to other carbs, they are definitely high in carbs and the slow absorption means the microbes get in on the action producing gas. Especially stay away from fruit juices which many times (apple and grape juice for instance) contain more sugar than sugar sweetened soft drinks. I tend to stay away from most fruits in general, but if I do consume fruits, I consume small amounts preferring to use them for garnishes. I use lime and lemon wedges in drinks and for cooking as well as to flavor prepared dishes like fish. I also use lemons, limes and oranges to add flavor when marinating meats. You don't need to consume a lot of fruit to get the benefits of their vitamins and minerals (and you will also be taking a multivitamin anyway). Fruits like strawberries and other berries have lower net carb counts and are the preferred fruits for low carbers. Just keep in mind the total net carb limits you are adhering to.

Fats

Fats are present in most foods that contain protein such as meats, fish, eggs, cheese and poultry listed above, but are also found in vegetable based oils like peanut and olive oil as well as in some vegetables like avocados. Remember from the discussion on fats in Chapter 4, our body does not produce omega-6- fatty acids and omega-3-fatty acids so these must be supplied in the diet. Since meats from grain fed animals provide ample omega-6-fatty acids you should just be concerned with including dietary sources of omega-3 fatty acids from foods such as fish and fish oil.

Stay away from trans-fats as much as possible. These are found in vegetable shortening, as well as vegetable oils like corn, sunflower, canola and flaxseed oil and even soybean oil because of the way these products are manufactured. Replace these products with olive, peanut, sesame or various nut-based oils as well as butter and fats from meats and poultry.

Snacks and Desserts

The constant proliferation of low carb dietary products offered by major food labels will help you a great deal in embracing a reduced carb lifestyle. Protein drinks have almost no carbs and provide a great pick-me-up between meals. Low carb brownies, cereal, cookies, ice cream are very tasty alternatives to high carb desserts. Lean towards desserts flavored with Splenda as opposed to sugar alcohols. Other foods I snack on include popcorn, baked mozzarella or parmesan cheese, mixed nuts, jerky and low carb sweets. If you want to bake your own sweets there are numerous low carb recipes available now (Low-carb Comfort Cook Book and Dana Carpenter's 15-Minute Low-Carb Recipes are a good place to start). And let's not forget about a low carb beer or glass of wine. After a while, it's hard to believe you are actually on any type of diet. Many of the foods do not sound low carb, but they are. Just be sure to read the labels to be sure about the net carb levels.

Do be careful about eating too many sweets made with high levels of sugar alcohols. Sugar alcohols are not absorbed and are eventually metabolized by your intestinal microbes. Though the gas from sugar alcohols is generally produced in the colon as opposed to the small intestine thus minimizing their impact on heartburn, they are associated with significant flatulence and will have a laxative effect over about 7 grams per serving. Snack bars and candies with too many sugar alcohols can rake havoc with you lower intestines. If you want to experiments with these products use moderation. Try one to three small candies or a half of a snack bar until you determine if your body can handle the sugar alcohols. I personally am very sensitive to sugar alcohols and try to avoid them as much as possible.

Complex vs. Simple Carbs

A general rule of thumb is that the more complex a carbohydrate is, the lower the glycemic index is. Low glycemic index foods are digested and absorbed more slowly thus having less impact on insulin levels (relating to the general health benefits of low carb dieting) and resulting in somewhat less gas production in the upper intestine compared to high glycemic index foods. It is the lower glycemic index foods that are the best overall choice for carbs that you add to your diet. The complex carbohydrate foods like nuts, whole grain breads, brown rice, beans and oatmeal generally have a lot of fiber that is healthy for your colon, and if consumed in moderation, will have less of an impact on heartburn. Remember that this is not a free pass on the carbohydrates. You will need to stick to your optimal overall level of carbohydrate intake that will likely be approximately one sixth of what you previously consumed on a high carb diet.

Comparing Net Carb Levels for Various Foods

Tables 2 through 11 list many foods from various food groups, the amount considered and the net carb level for that amount. These tables are intended to help you determine what foods and what amounts can be used in meal preparation in order to maintain your desired level of daily net carbs.

Table 2. Vegetables (Lower Carb)

Food	Amount	Net Carbs Per Serving (Grams)
alfalfa sprouts	1/2 cup	0.2
arugula	1/2 cup	0.4
asparagus	5 spears	3
bamboo shoots (canned)	1/2 cup	2.3
beans (snap)	1/2 cup	3.8
beans (wax)	1/2 cup	4.5
bok choy	1/2 cup	0.4
brussels sprouts	1/2 cup	5

Table 2. Vegetables (Lower Carb), continued

Food	Amount	Net Carbs Per Serving (Grams)
cabbage (green)	1/2 cup	2
cabbage (red)	1/2 cup	2
cauliflower	1/2 cup	2.7
celery	1 stalk	2
cucumber	1 each	5
endive	1/2 cup	0.8
green beans	1/2 cup	4
green chili	1 tbs	<1
lettuce	1/2 cup	0.6
mixed greens	1/2 cup	0.7
mushrooms (cooked)	1/2 cup	2.4
olives (black)	5 olives	1
olives (green)	3 each	1
onions (chopped)	1/2 cup	5
peppers (green)	1/2 cup	4
peppers (jalapenos)	1 each	<1
peppers (red)	1/2 cup	4
pickles (unsweetened)	1/2 large	1
popcorn (cooked)	1 cup	4

Table 2. Vegetables (Lower Carb), continued

Food	Amount	Net Carbs Per Serving (Grams)
pumpkin	1/2 cup	5
radishes	5 each	0.8
scallions	1/2 cup	2.5
snow peas	1/2 cup	4
spinach (cooked)	1/2 cup	2.5
spinach (uncooked)	1/2 cup	0.3
squash (spaghetti)	1/2 cup	5
squash (yellow)	1/2 cup	2.5
tomato (medium)	1 each	5
turnip	1/2 cup	4

Table 3. Vegetables (Higher Carb)

Food	Amount	Net Carbs Per Serving (Grams)
artichoke	1/2 cup	6
beets	1/2 cup	8
carrots	1/2 cup	6
chickpeas	1/2 cup	22
corn	1/2 cup	16
lentils	1/2 cup	20
peas	1/2 cup	10
potato (sweet)	1/2 each	11
potato (white)	1/2 each	10
soy beans	1/2 cup	10
squash (acorn)	1/2 cup	12
squash (butternut	1/2 cup	11
water chestnuts	1/2 cup	8
zucchini	1/2 cup	7

Table 4. Nuts

Food	Amount	Net Carbs Per Serving (Grams)
almonds	1/4 cup	6
cashews	1/4 cup	9
hazelnuts	1/4 cup	4
macadamias	1/4 cup	4
mixed nuts	1/4 cup	6
walnuts	1/4 cup	5
sunflower seeds	5 each	1
pistachios (no shells)	1/4 cup	6
pecans	1/4 cup	5
pine nuts	1/4 cup	4
peanuts	1/4 cup	5
sesame seeds	1/4 cup	7

Table 5. Breads, Cereals and Grains

Food	Amount	Net Carbs Per Serving (Grams)
bagel	1 each	30
biscuit	1 each	20
bread (Italian)	1 piece	15
bread (pita, small size)	1 each	33
bread (raisin)	1 piece	14
bread (rye)	1 piece	16
bread (sourdough)	1 piece	13
bread (wheat)	1 piece	12
bread (white)	1 piece	14
bread (whole grain)	1 piece	12
cereal (South Beach Diet Whole Grain Crunch)	3/4 cup	17
cereal (Special K Low Carb Lifestyle)	3/4 cup	9
cereal (Total Protein)	3/4 cup	7
cornmeal (whole-grain)	2 tbs	10
crackers (rye wafers)	1 each	9

Table 5. Breads, Cereals and Grains, continued

Food	Amount	Net Carbs Per Serving (Grams)
crackers (saltine, club, Ritz)	2 each	4
crackers (Triscuits)	2 each	6
croissant	1 each	24
English muffin	1 each	27
flour (stone ground whole wheat)	1/4 cup	21
flour (white)	1/4 cup	21
oat bran (raw)	2 tbs	6
oatmeal (plain, cooked)	1/2 cup	16.5
pancake (4 inch regular)	2 each	24
pancake (4 inch, low carb)	2 each	6
pasta (cooked)	1/2 cup	20
pasta (uncooked)	1 oz	21
pizza crust (thin crust 9 " diameter)	1/8 pizza	15
rice (brown, cooked)	1/2 cup	21
rice (brown, uncooked)	1/4 cup	29

Table 5. Breads, Cereals and Grains, continued

Food	Amount	Net Carbs Per Serving (Grams)
rice (white, cooked)	1/2 cup	22
rice (white, uncooked)	1/4 cup	35
rice (wild, cooked)	1/2 cup	17.5
sandwich roll	1 each	30
tortilla (corn)	1 each	12
tortilla (low carb, burrito size)	1 each	10
tortilla (low carb, fajita size)	1 each	5
tortillas (flour)	1 each	26
whole-grain oats (uncooked)	1/2 cup	29

Table 6. Dairy and Soy

Food	Amount	Net Carbs Per Serving (Grams)
butter	1 tbs	0
cheese (american)	1 slice	0.3
cheese (blue)	2 tbs	0.4
cheese (brie)	2 tbs	<1
cheese (cheddar)	2tbs	<1
cheese (cream)	1 oz	<1
cheese (goat)	2 tbs	0.3
cheese (jack)	1/4 cup	<1
cheese (muenster)	2 tbs	0.2
cheese (parmesan)	2 tbs	0
cheese (provolone)	1/2 cup	<1
cheese (ricotta, whole milk)	1/4 cup	2
cheese (swiss)	2 tbs	0.5
coffee mate	1 tsp	1
cottage cheese (whole milk)	1/2 cup	5
half and half	2 tbs	1
heavy cream	1/2 cup	3.5
ice cream (low carb)	1/2 cup	4
ice cream (normal)	1/2 cup	19
milk (2%)	1/2 cup	6

Table 6. Dairy and Soy, continued

Food	Amount	Net Carbs Per Serving (Grams)
plain yogurt (whole milk)	1/2 cup	6
sour cream	2 tbs	1
soy milk	1/2 cup	3.5
soy milk (unsweetened)	1/2 cup	2
tofu	4 oz	5

Table 7. Desserts

Food	Amount	Net Carbs Per Serving (Grams)
brownie mix (carb monitor)	1 each	13
brownie mix (regular)	1 each	24
cake (chocolate)	1 slice (2 oz)	26
cake (coffee)	1 slice (2 oz)	30
cake (pound)	1 slice (2 oz)	28
chocolate	1 oz	17

Table 7. Desserts, continued

Food	Amount	Net Carbs Per Serving (Grams)
cookie (chocolate chip)	1 each (1/2 oz)	11
cookie (oatmeal)	1 each (1/2 oz)	13
cookie (peanut butter)	1 each (1/2 oz)	9
cookie (sugar)	1 each (1/2 oz)	10
doughnut (glazed)	1 each	25
doughnut (plain)	1 each	20
ice cream (low carb)	1/2 cup	4
ice cream (normal)	1/2 cup	19
pie (apple)	1 piece (average)	60
pie (cherry)	1 piece (average)	70
pie (pecan)	1 piece (average)	65
pie (pumpkin)	1 piece (average)	40

Table 8. Drinks

Drinks	Amount	Net Carbs Per Serving (Grams)
beer (low carb)	12 oz	2.8
beer (regular)	12 oz	13
cola (diet)	12 oz	0
cola (regular)	12 oz	40
Crystal Light	12 oz	0
hard alcohols (non sweetened	1 oz	0
juice (apple)	1/2 cup	15
juice (cranberry)	1/2 cup	19
juice (grape)	1/2 cup	19
juice (grapefruit)	1/2 cup	11
juice (tomato)	1/2 cup	5
red wine (dry)	4 oz	2
Triple Sec liqueur	1 oz	12.5
white wine (dry)	4 oz	1

Table 9. Cooking, Baking

Food	Amount	Net Carbs Per Serving (Grams)
brownie mix (carb monitor)	1 each	13
brownie mix (regular)	1 each	24
chocolate chips	1 tbs	9
cocoa unsweetened	1 tbs	3
dressing (italian)	2 tbs	2
dressing (ranch)	2 tbs	2
dressing (thousand island)	2 tbs	5
heavy cream	1 cup	6.5
juice (lemon)	2 tbs	1.3
juice (lime)	2 tbs	1.4
ketchup	1 tbs	4
mayonaise	2 tbs	0
mustard	1 tbs	0
parmesan cheese	1/4 Cup	1
peanut butter	2 tbsp	2.5
salsa	2 tbs	2
scallions	1/4 Cup	1.2
sour cream	2 tbs	1
soy sauce	3 tbs	<1
sugar (brown)	1 tsp	4
sugar (white)	1 tsp	4

Table 9. Cooking, Baking, continued

Food	Amount	Net Carbs Per Serving (Grams)
tarter sauce	2 tbs	6
tomato sauce	1/2 cup	13

Table 10. Beans

Food	Amount	Net Carbs Per Serving (Grams)
beans (baked)	1/2 cup	28
beans (black)	1/2 cup	19
beans (lima)	1/2 cup	21
beans (navy)	1/2 cup	24
beans (pinto)	1/2 cup	22
beans (red kidney)	1/2 cup	20
beans (refried)	1/2 cup	18
chili (no bean)	1/2 cup	9
chili (with beans)	1/2 cup	16
hummus	2 tbs	6
Lentils	1/2 cup	20
peas (black eyed)	1/2 cup	18
soy beans	1/2 cup	10

Table 11. Fruits

Food	Amount	Net Carbs Per Serving (Grams)
apple	1/2 each	10
banana	1/2 each	10
blackberries	1/4 cup	2.9
blueberries	1/3 cup	5
boysenberries	1/2 cup	5
cantaloupe	1/4 each	10
cherries	5 each	4
cranberries (dried)	1/3 cup	33
dates	1 each	6
figs	1 each	10
grapefruit	1/2 each	9
grapes	1/2 cup	7.6
guava	1/2 each	5.3
kiwi	1 each	9
lemon	1 each	5
lime	1 each	7
mango	1/3 cup	10
orange	1/2 each	6
papaya	1/2 each	13
peach	1/2 each	5
pear	1/2 each	10
pineapple	1/2 cup	10

Table 11. Fruits, continued

Food	Amount	Net Carbs Per Serving (Grams)
plum (small)	1 each	7
prunes (dried)	1 each	5.3
raisons	1/4 cup	31
raspberries	1/2 cup	3
strawberries	1/2 cup	3.5
tangerine	1/2	5
watermelon	1/2 cup	5.5

Closing Remarks

As a GERD patient myself, and someone who suffered extensively with this condition for many years, I have enjoyed writing this book, because I know it will help many people who suffer with chronic heartburn. I hope you enjoy the information I have provided and will experience the relief I have by adopting a healthy life-long eating strategy that replaces excess carbs with more proteins and healthy fats.

Index

A

abdominal bloating, 32

acetate, 54, 64

acid reducers, 4-5

adenocarcinoma, 20

aerobic, 10

alcohol, 3, 6, 92-93, 107-108, 121

amines, 67

amino acid, 37, 40-45, 51-54, 66-67

ammonia, 67-68

amylopectin, 39

amylose, 39

anaerobic, 10, 61, 64

antacid, 4-5, 26

asthma, 18-22

B

Bacteroides fragilis, 12, 62

Bacteroides vulgatus, 62

bad breath, 18

barium, 17

Barrett's esophagus, 19-20

Bicarbonate, 26, 51, 69

Bifidobacterium sp., 62

Bile, 14, 16, 36, 51-54, 72-73, 88

blood pressure, 4, 47

bread, 37, 39, 100-103, 109, 115-117

bronchitis, 21

brush boarder, 52

butter, 43-46, 107, 113, 118-122

butyrate, 54, 64

C

Calcium, 46-47, 94, 96

Candy, 37, 82

canola oil, 44

carbon dioxide, 59, 68-69

carbonated soft drinks, 78-79

cecum, 53

cellulose, 39, 59

cheating, 4-5, 93, 99-101

children, 11, 20-23, 31

chyme, 50-53

chymotrypsin, 51

cigarettes, 92

cimetidine, 27-28

cisapride, 31

Clostridium perfringens, 62

coconut oil, 45

coffee, 3, 6, 8, 92, 118

colon, 40, 53-54, 63-64, 83, 108-109

confusion, 28

constipation, 28-29

cough, 5, 18, 21

cream, 45, 102, 118, 119, 122

D

dairy products, 37

death, 4, 31-32

dental erosion, 18

desserts, 92-93, 107, 120

diarrhea, 28-33

disaccharide, 38, 49, 81

dizziness, 28

duodenum, 14, 50-51, 63, 69-74

dysphagia, 19, 32-33

E

earache, 18

eicosanoids, 44

energy, 7, 10, 33, 37-43, 47, 52-54, 62, 65-66, 74, 92

Enterococcus faecalis, 62

erythromycin, 59-60

Escherichia coli, 62

esomeprazole, 28

esophageal cancer, 79-81

esophagoscopy, 17

esophagus, 5, 14-20, 26-27, 30-32, 48, 58, 60, 72-74, 80, 84, 89

essential amino acids, 41-42, 54

Eubacterium sp., 62

evolution, 71, 95

explosion (from intestinal gas), 69

F

famotidine, 27

fat, 4-11, 25, 33, 36-37, 40-46, 50-53, 57, 64-66, 68, 83, 86, 91-92, 94-95, 101-102, 104-107, 125

fatigue, 28

fatty acid, 37, 43-45, 51-54, 64, 66, 106-107

fecal, 54

fermentation, 10, 61, 64, 77, 87

fiber, 37, 39-40, 54, 64-65, 68-69, 93, 103-104, 109

flatulence, 33, 61, 83, 108

flatus, 67, 71-72, 83

flaxseed oil, 45, 107

flour, 37, 39, 103, 116-117

fructooligosaccharides, 77

fructose, 38, 40, 81

fruit juice, 81, 105

fuel, 38, 40, 89-90, 94

fundoplication, 23, 31, 32

fungi, 61

G

galactose, 38

gall bladder, 51

gas, 10-11, 17, 25, 32-33, 38, 54-62, 66-83, 89-96, 99, 105, 108, 109

gas-bloat syndrome, 60

gastric distension, 58, 79

gingivitis, 18

glucose, 36-41, 64, 69, 82

glycemic index, 81-83, 105, 109

grain, 37, 39-40, 43, 45, 105-106, 109, 115-117

H

H. pylori, 62

H2 blocker, 26-28

headache, 28-29

histamine, 27-31, 48

hydrochloric acid, 16, 27, 29

hydrogen, 38, 40, 43-44, 59, 68-70, 72, 77

hydrogen bond, 43

hydrogenation (trans-fats), 44, 46

I

ileum, 51, 53, 63

impotence, 28

insulin, 82, 93, 109

iron, 46, 47

J

jejunum, 51-52, 63, 65, 66

L

lactase, 51

Lactobacillus sp., 62

lactose, 38, 40, 65, 81

lactulose, 76-77

laparoscopy, 32

laxative, 108

lipase, 51, 66

liver, 51-52, 54

M

maintenance diet, 90, 98

malabsorption, 65, 76-77

maltase, 51

maltose, 51

meal plan, 12, 25

meteorism, 33

methane, 59, 68-70

Metoclopramide, 31

microbiology, 10

microvilli, 52

milk, 38, 81-82, 101-102, 118-119

minerals, 37, 46-47, 106

monosaccharide, 38, 51-52, 82-83

monounsaturated fats, 44

motilin-like (effect), 59

mouth, 15, 47

mucus, 48-49

muscle, 15, 17, 41, 48, 50, 54, 56, 58-59, 70, 75, 98

N

nausea, 29, 31

nervous system effects, 31

Nexium, 25, 28

Nissen Fundoplication, 31, 32

nitrates, 102

nitrogen, 40-41, 67

nutrient absorption, 52, 64-65, 83

nutrients, 9-10, 37, 51-54, 61-65, 83

O

olive oil, 44, 106

omega-3 fatty acid, 45, 107

omega-6 fatty acid, 45

omeprazole, 28

osmotic balance, 47

oxygen, 10, 38, 40, 43, 61-62, 64, 66

P

palm oil, 45

pancreas, 51

peanut oil, 44

parietal cells, 27-28, 48

Pepcid, 27

pepsin, 26, 50

peptide bond, 42

peristalsis, 15, 59, 73

pH, 17, 22, 26, 47-49, 67-68

pneumonia, 4, 29-30

phosphorus, 46

polypeptide, 50-51

polysaccharide, 38-39, 49-51

polyunsaturated fats, 44-45

portal vein, 52

postnasal drip, 18

Prilosec, 28

prokinetic agents, 31

promotility agents, 31

protein, 4, 7, 9-11, 26, 36-37, 40-43, 46, 50-52, 57, 59, 64-68, 83, 91-95, 101-102, 105-106, 125

proton pump inhibitors, 28-29, 31

protozoa, 61

propionate, 54, 64

putrefaction, 66

pyloric sphincter, 50, 71, 72

R

ranitidine, 27

regurgitation, 14, 18, 21

respiration, 10

S

safflower (oil), 45

saliva, 47, 49

salt, 47, 53, 92

satiety, 33

saturated fats, 44-45

side effects, 4, 22, 24, 28-29, 31

smoking, 3

snacks, 100-101, 105, 107

Splenda, 92, 104, 107

starch, 37-40, 47, 50, 69, 81, 103-105

stomach, 3, 5, 14-17, 20, 26-33, 47-51, 58-63, 67-74, 79-80, 83, 89

stomach bloating, 58

Streptococcus sp., 62

stress, 92

stricture, 19

sucrase, 51

sucrose, 38, 40

sugar, 37-41, 43, 47, 49, 68-70, 80-82, 87, 92-93, 103, 106-108, 120, 122

sugar alcohols, 93, 107-108

sulfur, 40-41

surgery, 11, 21-22, 31-33, 47, 60-61, 69

T

table sugar, 38

Tagamet, 27

trans-fats, 44, 46, 92, 107

triglycerides, 50-51

trypsin, 51

V

vegetable oil, 43, 46, 107

vegetables, 37, 43, 102-106, 110-113

villi, 52

viruses, 61

vitamins, 9, 37, 46, 53-54, 61, 105-106

W

water, 37, 46-47, 53-54, 64, 79, 94

western diet, 95

X

X-rays, 17

Z

Zantac, 27

Zoton, 28